GRAD (Gravitational Resistance And Diet) System

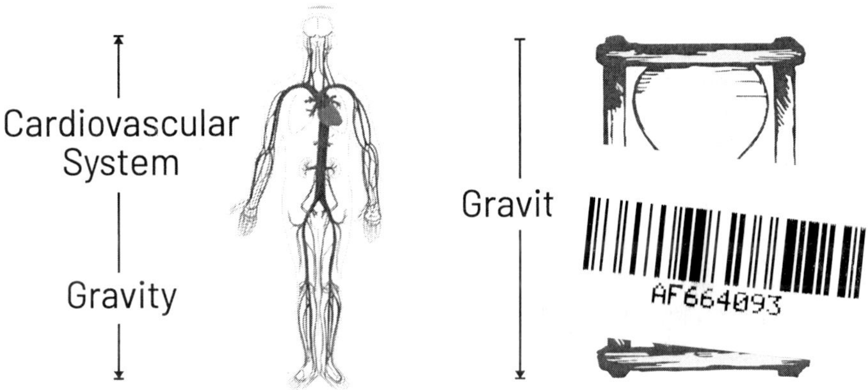

A Sand Clock, also known as an Hour Glass, works on the basic force of gravity. Similarly, human body also works on the same force of gravity where instead of sand, we have blood in the veins. In addition to the force of gravity, the body also has the force of pressure generated by the cardiovascular system (not just the heart) that controls the flow of all body fluids including blood. The balance between these two forces controls various aspects of our body, which includes our physical and mental health (for further details, read the book "360° Postural Medicine"). GRAD system can be seen as first-ever scientifically validated tool to re-establish the lost balance of the body. It achieves the goal to reverse life-threatening medical conditions, including Diabetes, Hypertension, and Chronic Kidney Diseases, using the gravitational force.

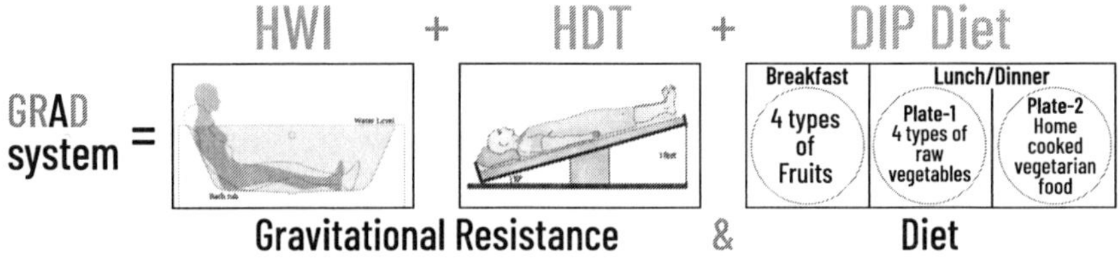

End of Transplant

India Office:
C/o India Book of Records
B-121, 2nd Floor, Greenfields,
Faridabad -120003 (Haryana),
India
Ph.: +91-9312286540

Malaysia Office:
C/o Bishwaroop International Healing & Research
PT 573, Lot 15077 Jalan Tuanku
Munawir,
70000 Negeri Sembilan, Malaysia
Tel: +6012-2116089

Vietnam Office:
C/o Vietnam Book of Records
148 Hong Ha Street
9 Award, Phu Nhuan District,
Ho Chi Minh City, Vietnam
- Hotline: (+84) 903710505

Switzerland Office:
C/o Nigel Kingsley
Kraftwerkstr. 95, ch-5465, Mellikon,
Switzerland
Tel: 0041 79 222 2323

FOLLOW ME

Youtube: https://www.youtube.com/c/NICEupdates
Facebook: https://www.facebook.com/ivmb.official
Twitter: https://www.twitter.com/CoronakaalT
Bitchute: https://www.bitchute.com/channel/drbiswarooproychowdhury
Telegram: https://t.me/drbiswarooproychowdhury
Email: biswaroop@biswaroop.com
Website: www.biswaroop.com
Video Channel: www.coronakaal.tv

Research: Rachna Sharma
GRAD Team: Kalpana Bourai, Dr. Indupreet Kaur
Transcription: Divya Tiwari
Graphic Design: Swapan Banik

Diamond Pocket Books
X-30, Okhla Industrial Area, New Delhi-110020
Ph: 011-40712100 email: sales@dpb.in website: www.diamondbook.in

Dedication

To all the patients, for showing unflinching faith in GRAD system. By adopting the GRAD System, they have set an example for the First time in the world that Chronic Kidney Disease is reversible and Kidney Transplant is avoidable.

Disclaimer

1. GRAD System is not approved by any government body. One may follow it in good faith with a promise not to go for litigation under any circumstances.
2. Medicine/hospital related advise is entirely patient's decision/call.

Contents

Foreword

Gravitational Resistance and Diet (GRAD) System is developed by Dr. Biswaroop Roy Chowdhury for reversing Chronic Kidney Disease (CKD). Thousands of CKD patients are benefiting by this treatment protocol and several hospitals have already adopted the GRAD System. Shridhar University in collaboration with Dayanand Ayurvedic College conducted an observational study to find the effectiveness of GRAD System. The study concluded that among the patients who adopted the GRAD system completely 75% could free themselves of dialysis and 89% could free themselves of full or partial dependence on drugs.

Hence, GRAD System is the only known scientifically validated method to reverse Chronic Kidney Disease.

This book is divided in two sections.

Section-I is the **"Prospective Cohort Study on GRAD System"**, which will enable a layman, a doctor, and patient's caretakers to get answers to the following questions:

1. How to implement GRAD System to reverse CKD?
2. How many days of following GRAD System can help a CKD patient get freedom from dependence on dialysis and drugs?
3. What are the chances of reversal of CKD by following GRAD System?

Section-II deals with Frequently Asked Questions and important instructions for CKD patients who are following the GRAD System.

This book can be seen as the beginning of the **'End of Transplant'** era.

Section - I

Prospective Cohort Study

Effectiveness of Gravitational Resistance and Diet (GRAD) system in reversing Chronic Kidney Disease (CKD) - among dialysis patients.

- Dr. Awadhesh Pandey (Department of Medical Sciences, Shridhar University, Pilani, Rajasthan, India)
- Dr. Amar Singh Azad (Department of Medical Sciences, Shridhar University, Pilani, Rajasthan, India)
- Dr. Anu Bhardwaj, (Department of Medical Sciences, Shridhar University, Pilani, Rajasthan, India)
- Dr. Gagan Thakur, (Dayanand Ayurvedic College, Jalandhar, Punjab, India)
- Dr. Gayathri M Prakash, (Dayanand Ayurvedic College, Jalandhar, Punjab, India)

Highlights:

1. The pioneering cohort study to assess the effectiveness of GRAD system in reversing CKD among dialysis patients.
2. Gravitational resistance and DIP diet[1] were utilized in the GRAD System as the main tools to help patients reverse CKD (Chronic Kidney Disease).
3. Head Down Tilt (HDT) and Hot Water Immersion (HWI) were used to induce gravitational resistance[2].
4. 100 Dialysis patients formed the sample study group and were assessed and recorded on a variety of parameters for an average of 100 days.

5. Among the patients who adopted GRAD system fully, 75% were relieved from having to undergo Dialysis and 89% could free themselves of full or partial dependence on drugs.
6. Quality of life improved and economic burden reduced among 92% of the patients who followed the GRAD System.

ABSTRACT

BACKGROUND: The global prevalence of Chronic Kidney Disease (CKD) ***referred to as mutraghat/mutrakshay*** in Ayurveda is nearly 70 crores[3], with nearly 1/3rd of the patients belonging to either India or China. There has been no lasting and effective cure till now, and the only available treatments are either Dialysis or Kidney transplants.

OBJECTIVE: The objective of the Study was to determine the effectiveness of the GRAD System developed by Dr. Biswaroop Roy Chowdhury in reversing CKD among the patients who are dependent on Dialysis.

METHODS: This was a prospective cohort study conducted from August 2021 to March 2022. 100 dialysis patients, who agreed to adopt GRAD system in their lifestyle for an average of 100 days were closely monitored and data on various parameters carefully recorded. Data was collected using interviewer-administered questionnaires, examination of participants, and review of medical records.

RESULTS: 28 out of 100 dialysis patients fully adopted the GRAD system. Among them, 21 (75%) were completely free of dialysis and supporting drugs while the remaining 25% were partially free of dialysis and supporting drugs.

72 patients partially adopted the GRAD system. Among them, 11 (15%) were able to be free of all the supporting drugs while 44 could reduce the frequency of dialysis. Quality of life improved among 100% of the patients and their economic burden reduced from 70% to 90% in 58% of the patients. There was no serious negative impact seen and no death or adverse event was reported as a result of the adherence to GRAD System. In fact, all the patients experienced a marked improvement in their health, spirits and financial well-being.

CONCLUSION: GRAD system can be recommended as an effective method to reverse CKD among mild, moderate, and severe CKD patients and can be seen as an effective alternative to dialysis and kidney transplant.

Received: March 21, 2022, Accepted: March 29, 2022

Competing Interests: The authors have declared no competing interests.

Introduction

Chronic Kidney Disease (CKD) ***refered to as mutraghat*[4] *mutrakshay*** in Ayurveda is a lasting condition all over the globe.

Kidneys don't work as they should. It's a common condition associated with getting older. Moreover, the person on allopathic medications of hypertension, their kidneys are damaged in the long run. So mostly people on allopathic drugs develop CKD and finally turn into dialysis patients due to side effects and the over medications showing the effects on the kidneys[5].The economic as well as the social life of the relatives of the patients is also affecting. The cost of living of the dialysis patients is higher[6].

Until now, there had been no known intervention scientifically proven to help severe CKD patients to reverse the disease and free themselves of their dependency on dialysis, transplant and drugs. However, in the modern scientific literature, there are references of Head Down Tilt (HDT) and Hot Water Immersion (HWI) which are known to activate the kidney. These techniques can also effectively excrete Sodium by five times, Potassium by three times, increase the urine volume by three times and result in the overall reduction of body weight and swelling[7]. Even in Ayurveda, there are several references of HWI referred to as Avagaha SWED[8] as an effective method to rejuvenate the compromised kidneys.

Need for the Study

Chronic Kidney disease (CKD) is a progressive, irreversible decline in renal function that occurs over time. The only symptom is a metabolic anomaly at first. When the glomerular filtration rate (GFR) falls below 30 ml/min, CKD is evaluated. The traditional management method comprises dialysis and kidney transplantation, both of which are out of reach for the Indian populace due to financial constraints. As a result, research into a safe and alternative therapy that can assist reduce the need for dialysis and delay or stop the need for kidney transplantation is required.

An average kidney transplant costs Rs 2,00,000 in a government hospital and Rs 7,00,000 to 10,00,000 in a private facility. In addition, the annual medicine maintenance cost after the transplant is Rs 2,00,000 per year or Rs 20,000 per month. As a result, the social and economic ramifications of CKD are significant, and the traditional therapeutic method comprises dialysis and kidney transplantation, both of which are unaffordable and unacceptable to the Indian people. Research into a safe and alternative therapy that can assist reduce the need for dialysis and delay the need for kidney transplantation is critical. Several institutes and academics are attempting to make progress in this approach.

Dr Biswaroop Roy Chowdhury combined HDT, HWI and the DIP diet to develop a protocol called the GRAD System, with the goal to reverse kidney failure, especially among the patients who are dialysis dependent.

Objectives and Goals of the Study

- To demonstrate the effectiveness of the combination of various techniques and Ayurvedic remedies in the treatment of CKD.
- To provide a future therapeutic option for a large human population suffering from CKD, with the goal of minimising the need for dialysis and avoiding or delaying kidney transplantation.

Methods and Techniques

2 hours of HDT + 2 hours of HWI + DIP Diet = GRAD System. As part of the GRAD system, dialysis patients are encouraged to do 2 hours of HDT and HWI every day along with following the DIP Diet. Every day for the purpose of monitoring the patient's P R A N (Patients Reporting to Activate Nephrons) sheet is being maintained for each of the patients through the GRAD app. In PRAN sheet following parameters are being monitored.

Weekly P R A N Sheet (For Kidney / Liver Patients) Arrow represents the expected outcome of the patients on GRAD system						
Date	B.P.	Pulse ↔	↓ Weight	↓ Swelling (yes/no)	↑ Urine Output (If <400 ML)	↓ Symptoms
1	HDT	HDT	HWI	HDT		
	1. 2.	1. 2.	1. 2.	1. 2.		
	HWI ↓	HWI	HWI	HWI		
	3. 4.	3. 4.	3. 4.	3. 4.		

Based on the improvement on the above parameters, the patients who participated in the study were required to taper down or phase out the drugs and various other medications which they were taking and to reduce the frequency of dialysis. Patients were advised to gradually increase the duration of HDT / HWI as the body adapted to the therapies and started showing positive improvement. Many patients could adhere to the GRAD system partially because of poor family support, lack of discipline or because of discouragement from their dialysis centers or other reasons.

What is Head Down Tilt (HDT)[7]

When a patient is made to lie down at 10 degrees angle of the head, it leads to a decrease in the Plasma Aldosterone and Renin hormones in the body. This results in a decrease in Plasma volume and subsequently, an increase sodium excretion from the body.

HDT 10°

HDT > 5°

↓

Decrease in Plasma Aldosterone

\+

Plasma Renin

↓

Decrease in plasma volume

\+

Increase in sodium excretion

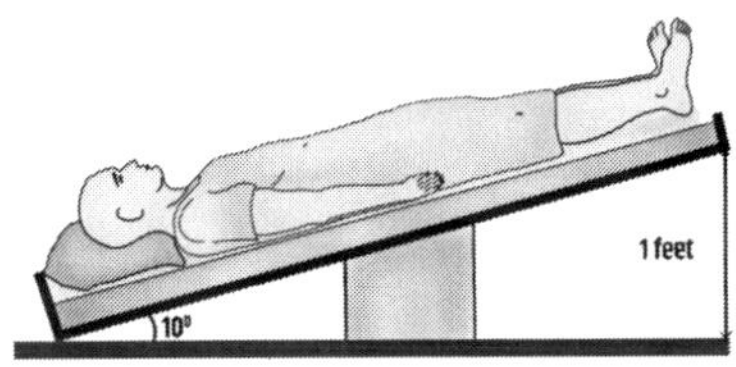

What is Hot Water Immersion HWI (Avagaha Swed)[8]

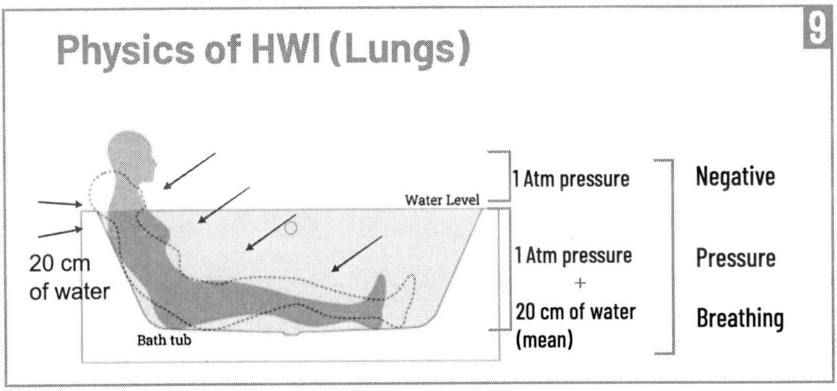

The Physics of HWI (Lungs)[9]

When a patient is made to sit in the bath tub with water level up to the neck, the air pressure above the neck is 1 Atmosphere. Below the neck the atmospheric pressure is 1 Atmosphere. If the mean height of the water in the bath tub is 20 cm, the pressure below the neck increases by about 2% (1 atm + 20 cm).

Therefore, when a patient sits in neck deep water, his body undergoes two different pressures, one above the neck and one below the neck. This difference in pressure results in negative pressure breathing.

10

Physics of HWI (Heart)

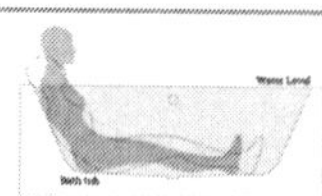

Stroke volume increase by 20%

+

Redistribution of blood from lower portion of body to intra-thoracic (middle) circulation

As a result of this breathing, a 20% increase in the stroke volume of the heart is observed. The heart pumps an increased volume of blood by 20% due to the negative pressure breathing.

This increased blood pumping leads to redistribution of blood from the lower portion of the body to the upper torso, waist upwards.

Chemistry of HWI[11]

As shown in image-11, the movement of the blood from being centred on the kidney upwards results in certain chemical changes in the body. The levels of IL-6, Ilira, Hsp72, 1Hsp72, and NO increase in the body whereas the levels of Norepinephrine, Vasopressin, and Renin decrease in the body within two hours of immersion of the body in the bath tub.

11

Chemistry of HWI

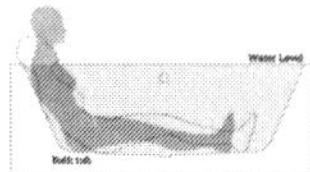

↑ Increase	↓ Decrease
IL-6, Ilira	Norepinephrine
Hsp72 , iHsp72	Vasopressin
NO	Renin

HWI Causes Dialysis [12]

12

HWI Causes Dialysis

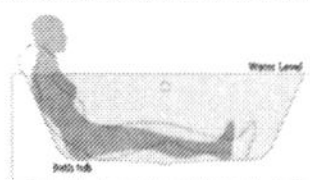

- Sodium Excretion 5 Times
- Potassium excretion doubles
- Urine volume increases three times
- Weight/swelling reduced

What is D.I.P. Diet

The D.I.P. (Disciplined and Intelligent diet) is being developed by Dr Biswaroop Roy Chowdhury and through clinical trials[1] and various case studies[13], it has been proven to be effective in reversing life style diseases.

Steps to Design Your Personalized D.I.P. Diet:

Step-I

Till 12:00 noon, eat only fruits of three to four types including mango, banana, grapes, etc.

Minimum amount to be consumed = Your body weight in kg × 10 = ___ gm

For example, a 70 kg person should consume at least 700 gm of 4 types of fruits before 12 noon.

Step-II

Always eat your lunch/dinner in two plates. Plate 1 and Plate 2.

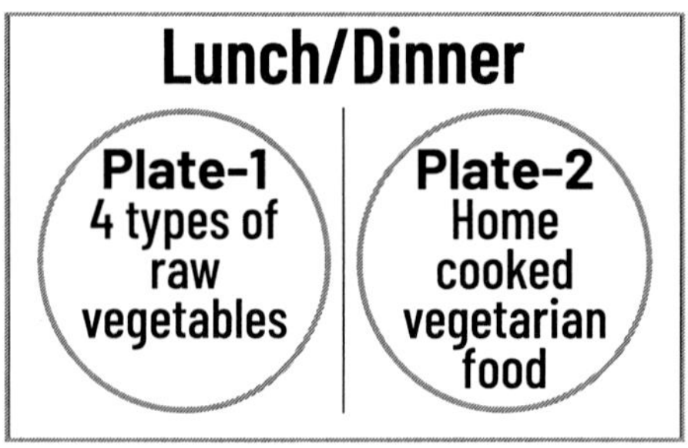

Plate 1 should consist of four types of vegetables like carrot, tomato, radish and cucumber etc. in raw form. Minimum amount in Plate 1 = Your body weight in kg × 5 =___ gm.

For example, a 70 kg person should eat at least 350 gm of four types of raw vegetables. Plate 2 should consist of home cooked vegetarian food with negligible salt and oil. (Replace wheat & rice with millets)

First finish eating from plate 1 in accordance with the above calculation, then take from plate 2 as much as you want. The rules for lunch and dinner are the same; however, you must remember to finish dinner by 7:00 P.M.

To Avoid	Snacking / Binge eating
1. Packed food	1. Soaked nuts: Your wt (kg) = __ gm (eg. 70 kg person can consume 70 gm of nuts in a day)
2. Refined food	2. Fruits: Plenty
3. Dairy food/Animal foods	3. Coconut water: As you like
4. Nutritional supplements	4. Sprouts: Your Wt.(kg) = __ gm
5. Avoid drinking tea/coffee specially before lunch	5. Coconut: As you like
6. Never eat after 8:00 P.M.	6. Sunshine: 45 min
7. NSAIDs	

Ayurvedic perspective of CKD and Hot Water Immersion (HWI)

Vrukk[14] or Kidneys in Ayurveda

Nirukti "वर्षति इति वक्: क" (अमरकोष)

The word derived from the word "वषृ सेचने" which means Irrigation.

"बकु " word is also used for vrukka (अमरकोष).

Functions "वृक्कौ पुष्टिकरौ प्रक्तौ जठरस्थस्य मेदस"

The human body and its nutritional element which is food or both derived from a combination of 5 elements (*Mahabhutas*). The various permutations and combinations of these five foundational elements of food and the body can be modified adapted or incorporated or eliminated to cause remedy or prevent certain conditions from arriving in arising in the body. This can then be transformed as *sajitha* or tissue in which specific substances or *Dutt wahrasa* (specific nutrients) can be incorporated for boosting *sharir dhaatus*.

Vrukk or Kidney is made up by *rakht* and *meda*, and is the end part of *Ahaarpaak*. The anatomical *Vrukk* is an organ and can be used to refer to the Renals, Suprarenals, Ureters and bladder in different contexts. Vrukk is the supplementary organ of *koshtha* and are located in the *koshtha*. *Vrukk* (Kidneys) and *Mutra Vaha Strotas* (Urinary Tract) or Nephrons are micro channels for the production and storage of urine.

Pathogenesis (Samprapti) of CKD / Mutraghat in Ayurveda

According to Ayurveda chronic kidney disease resemble with Mutraghat/ Aama in Mutra vaha Strotas. Ama in mutravaha strotas that hampers the function of kidney. Dosha Vata and Kapha mainly involved in it.[15]

Mutraghata

Mutra-Kshaya Dehydrated and Fatigued

Pathogenesis:- Even though a Ruksha person has no Pitta aggravating factors, but Pitta along with Vata has been stressed upon. This leads to still the involvement of the drying up of the urine.[16]

Mutrashoshana[17] – Clinical features: burning micturation, painful micturition, troublesome small quantity of urine.

Treatment of Vrukk Dosha mentioned in Charak and Susruta Samhita

Avagaha Sweda

Ayurvedic therapy or its incorporation or combination with other kind of therapies is primarily aimed and the maintenance of the **Homeostasis** in the system by eliminating the excess or undesirable elements and aiding in the absorption of the essential elements by the body.

Charak Samhita mentions the inclusion of Avagaha sweda as an effective treatment.

वातहरोत्क्वाथक्षीरतैलघृतपिशितरसोष्णसलिलकोष्ठकावगाहस्तु यथोक्त एवावगाहः||४५||

VataharotkvAthakShIratailaghRutapishitarasoShNasalilakoShThakAvagAhastu yathokta evAvagAhaH

Fomentation by immersion in a tub filled up with ***vata*** alleviating decoctions, milk, oil, ghee, meat juices or hot water is termed as ***avagaha***.

Sutra Sthana Chapter 14

Indications of *swedana*

प्रतिश्याये च कासे च हिक्काश्वासेष्वलाघवे| कर्णमन्याशिरःशूले स्वरभेदे गलग्रहे||२०||
अर्दितैकाङ्गसर्वाङ्गपक्षाघाते विनामके| कोष्ठानाहविबन्धेषु मूत्राघाते विजृम्भके||२१||
पार्श्वपृष्ठकटीकुक्षिसङ्ग्रहे गृध्रसीषु च| मूत्रकृच्छ्रे महत्त्वे च मुष्कयोरङ्गमर्दके||२२||
पादजानूरुजङ्घार्तिसङ्ग्रहे श्वयथावपि| खल्लीष्वामेषु शीते च वेपथौ वातकण्टके||२३||
सङ्कोचायामशूलेषु स्तम्भगौरवसुप्तिषु | सर्वाङ्गेषु विकारेषु स्वेदनं हितमुच्यते||२४||

It is said that *swedana* is useful in rhinitis, cough, hiccups, breathing difficulties, heaviness of body, earache, headache, cervical pain, hoarseness of voice, choking sensation of throat, facial palsy, monoplegia, quadriplegia, hemiplegia, prostrated postures, abdominal flatulence, constipation, urinary retention, excessive yawning, stiffness of flanks, dorsum, lumbar and abdomen, sciatica, dysuria, scrotal enlargement, body ache, pain and stiffness of dorsum of foot, knee, thigh and calf, edema, severely painful radiculopathy, indigestion, chills and shivering, subluxation of ankle, contractures, convulsions, colicky pains, stiffness, heaviness and numbness, and such disorders anywhere in the body.

सङ्करः प्रस्तरो नाडी परिषेकोऽवगाहनम्| जेन्ताकोऽश्मघनः कर्षूः कुटी भूः कुम्भिकैव च||३९||
कूपो होलाक इत्येते स्वेदयन्ति त्रयोदश| तान् यथावत् प्रवक्ष्यामि सर्वानेवानुपूर्वशः||४०||

Thirteen varieties of fomentation are *sankara, prastara, nadi, parisheka, avagahana, jentaka, ashmaghna, karshu, kuti, bhu, kumbhika, kupa,* and *holaka.* They are further detailed accordingly in the same sequence. [39-4]

The 13 varieties of Saagni Sweda include Avagaha.

Avagaha *swedana/Sudation* is classified as Saagni Sweda because it uses heated fluids that have been prepared with medicines only after coming into touch with heat or fire (by heating or boiling on fire).

Material for *Avagaha Wweda* (Tub Fomentation)

एत एव च निर्यूहाः प्रयोज्या जलकोष्ठके| स्वेदनार्थं घृतक्षीरतैलकोष्ठांश्च कारयेत्||३४||

These same decoctions can be used in a water tub for fomentation. In a similar manner, ghee, milk, and sesame oil may also be used in tub fomentation.

Abhyanga (herbal oil massage) with *Vatahara tailas* is administered to the individual (patient) who would get *Avagaha Sweda* (oils which alleviate vitiated vata). Later, he is forced to sit in a large tub that is large enough to fit him. He should sit in the tub with his neck and head above the water's surface. Fill the tub halfway with hot *vatahara dravas* (liquids having vata alleviating property). These liquids might be any of the following:

Vatahara Patra Kwatha — water-based decoctions created by ingesting and processing leaves with *vata*-relieving properties.

Vatahara Siddha Ksheera is milk that has been treated with *vata*-relieving decoctions.

Taila is a kind of oil that is used to treat a variety of ailments.

Ghrita is ghee that has been medicated.

Mamsarasa is a kind of soup.

Ushnodaka – warm water, and so on

Here in this study warm water was used for giving HWI

Avagaha sweda can also be made using *Siddha Jala* – water that has been prepared with herbs. This decoction is not made the usual way; instead, the water is just boiled with the herbs.

Duration of Time

According to the necessity and condition, *Avagaha Kala - Avagaha Sweda* should be administered for 1 *muhurta* (48 minutes) to 4 *muhurta* (192 minutes). Alternatively, sudation should be performed until the patient begins to sweat appropriately and exhibits signs and symptoms of proper *swedana*, as per the basic concept of *Swedana*.

Practise of HWI or Avgaha Sveda in History[18,19]

Hot water Immersion has always been an inherent part of daily life in almost all parts of the world. The practice of immersing in water has been such a fundamental ritual that it has even permeated into the daily lives of people as a ritual, spiritual exercise, stress busting technique, sanitary and hygienic practice etc. and also has been imbibed in a daily ritual and practices as part of religious rituals.

Historical references indicate that Hot Water treatment has been an inherent part of Indian as well as European culture since times immemorial. It has been prevalent in nations, cultures and almost all ancient civilizations have the tradition of having a communal bath in which people use to go and immerse themselves in Hot, Cold or normal water. This is true of the Indus valley civilization where the Great Bath at Mohenjo-daro and at all significant other sites are notable examples. The Sumerian civilization, Egyptian civilization as well as the Greek and Roman civilizations attached great importance to the bathing rituals.

In Ayurveda also, HWI treatment or Avagaha sweda has been prevalent in India since ancient times as evidenced by the finding of communal baths which have existed down the ages. Almost all the cities of the Harappan civilization, Ancient Rome, Babylon, Greece or Egypt and Persian Civilizations had Communal Baths or *Hamams* that have been frequently in use in Europe from ancient times to the medieval ages. Bathing in hot tubs was an important weekly ritual done before going to church on Sunday for the sanitary and health related benefits.

In India, this practice was incorporated in Ayurveda as Avagaha, sweda.

Study Site and Participants

GRAD study on Dialysis patients is a prospective cohort study on the patients who are currently reliant on dialysis. 100 Dialysis patients from across the country, who adopted the GRAD system (either fully or partially) were observed for an average 100 days from August 2021 to March 2022. 24% of the patients visited the Hospital and Institute of Integrated Medical Sciences (HIIMS) located in multiple locations of Dera Bassi, Punjab and Jaipur / Jodhpur, Rajasthan along with their family members to get the training on the GRAD System. The remaining 76% patients underwent online training through videos on implementing the GRAD System at home. 100 patients were located across 22 states with majority of the patients belonging to Delhi, Punjab, Haryana, and Rajasthan.

Inclusion criteria:

1. Patients who were on dialysis at least once a week.
2. Patients who were willing to adopt the GRAD System.

Exclusion criteria:

1. Patients not on dialysis.
2. Patients who discontinued following the GRAD system.

3. Patients who did not cooperate to share their daily progress report in accordance to PRAN sheet.

Data Collection

1. At the selection stage, patients were asked to fill the Diet and Medication (DAM) form and submit all relevant medical reports including KFT, 3 days of Blood pressure and blood sugar (if diabetes patients) and other relevant blood reports.
2. Subsequently, daily/weekly data were collected in accordance with the PRAN sheet. Various modes were used to monitor and collect the data, including telephonic calls, video conferencing, and also through a customized GRAD App. In addition to the PRAN sheet, the following information was also collected:

Weakness Scale (0-10)
Vomiting
Itching
Delirium
Seizure
Expenses (Dialysis / Care Taker / Medicines / Transport / Doctor)
Which Date Dialysis Stopped
Which Date Stopped Partially
Since When Medicines Stopped Partially
Since When Medicines Stopped Completely
Would you recommend this to others?

During the entire period of study, the patients were motivated to follow the GRAD system as closely and accurately as possible. They were also encouraged to share the relevant data including daily urine output, blood pressure, weight and any discomfort/symptoms on real time basis either through GRAD App or through telephonic conversation.

Evaluation of Study Participants

Trained research assistants obtained informed consent before participants were enrolled into the study. Demographic information was collected through interviews, and responses were collated and assessed on a questionnaire. This included age, gender, education, employment status along with lifestyle behaviors such as alcohol use, cigarette smoking, physical activity levels, frequency and quantity of daily fruit and vegetable consumption, and table salt intake. A detailed medical history including duration of CKD diagnosis and doses of medications being taken at the beginning of the study were also obtained.

Representation of the demographic profile of the patient group under study

Age	Gender		Total
	Female	Male	
15-20	2	2	4
20-25	1	3	4
25-30	3	1	4
30-35	2	3	5
35-40	4	9	13
40-45	5	14	19
45-50	7	7	14
50-55	3	6	9
55-60	3	5	8
60-65	1	2	3
65-70	1	9	10
70-75	2	0	2
75 above	1	4	5

Anthropometric evaluations including measurement of weight and height were recorded. Body Mass Index (BMI) of each participant was then derived by dividing the weight and height in meters.

Ethics Statement

The participants submitted informed consent in writing expressing their willingness to participate and adopt GRAD System. In the case of minors (04), their guardians and caretakers signed the consent form. Withdrawal from the study never jeopardized the participants' health.

Data Analysis

Data of 100 eligible patients was collected with an average monitoring duration being 100 days. The data is divided in 2 groups:

Group 1: Patients who followed GRAD system fully

Criteria of 100% adherence to GRAD system:

- 4 hours of HDT + HWI for more than 80% of the monitoring days.
- Following 100% DIP diet for more than 90% of the monitoring days.

Group 2: Criteria of partial adherence to GRAD system:

- 4 hours of HDT + HWI for less than 80% but more than 50% of the monitoring days.
- Following 100% DIP diet for less than 90% but more than 50% of the monitoring days.

Based on the above criteria only 28 participants were eligible in group 1 and 72 participants were eligible in group 2.

Patients adhering less than 50% or less of the time in HDT + HWI and less than 50% on DIP Diet were excluded from the study.

Representation of the Patients who witnessed improvement in passing of Urine as a result of adherence to the GRAD system

Effect on Urine	Frequency	Percent	Cum.
More	43	43.00	43.00
Same	39	39.00	82.00
Reduced	18	18.00	100.00
Total	**100**	**100.00**	

Correlation tested

To test if those who followed GRAD fully exhibited greater improvement than among those who followed it partially.

	Urine	
GRAD	**Increased**	**Total**
Fully	13 (46%)	28
Partially	30 (42%)	72
Total	**43 (43%)**	**100**

The group following GRAD fully have shown higher improvement in urination.

Representation of the Patients who witnessed improvement in incidence of swelling as a result of adherence to the GRAD system

Effect on Swelling	Frequency	Percent	Cum
Never existed	36	36.00	36.00
Swelling eliminated	23	23.00	59.00
Improved	18	18.00	77.00
Same	13	13.00	90.00
Deteriorated	10	10.00	100.00

Correlation tested

Swelling		
GRAD	**Reduced/eliminated**	**Total**
Fully	16 (57%)	28
Partially	24 (33%)	72
Total	**40 (40%)**	**100**

It can be clearly seen that the subjects who followed GRAD fully exhibited higher improvement in swelling (in terms of both reduction or elimination of swelling).

Representation of the impact on the weakness of patients as a result of adherence to the GRAD system

Effect on Weakness	Frequency	Percent	Cum
Reduced	47	47.00	47.00
Increased	24	24.00	71.00
No weakness ever reported	16	16.00	87.00
Same	13	13.00	100.00

Correlation tested

Weakness		
GRAD	**Reduced**	**Total**
Fully	15 (54%)	28
Partially	32 (44%)	72
Total	**47 (47%)**	**100**

The group following GRAD fully have shown higher improvement in reduction of weakness as compared to those who followed it partially.

Representation of the impact on the Breathlessness of patients as a result of adherence to the GRAD system

Effect on Breathlessness	Frequency	Percent	Cum
No breathlessness	47	47.00	47.00
Reduced	33	33.00	80.00
Increased	16	16.00	96.00
Same	4	4.00	100.00
Total	**100**	**100.00**	

Correlation tested

	Breathlessness	
GRAD	**Reduced**	**Total**
Fully	9 (32%)	28
Partially	24 (33%)	72
Total	**33 (33%)**	**100**

The group following GRAD fully seems to show lesser improvement in breathlessness than the partial group. However, this difference is not statistically significant. Thus we can conclude, there exists no difference in the percentage improvement shown by these two groups.

Representation of the impact on the dependence on Dialysis of patients as a result of adherence to the GRAD system

Effect on Dialysis	Frequency	Percent	Cum
Reduced	49	49.00	49.00
Same	28	28.00	77.00
Stopped	21	21.00	98.00
Ambiguous	2	2.00	100.00
Total	**100**	**100**	

Correlation tested

Dialysis		
GRAD	**Improvement**	**Total**
Fully	21 (75%)	28
Partially	49 (49%)	72
Total	**70 (70%)**	**100**

Significantly Higher improvement among the fully following group.

Representation of the Patients who witnessed improvement in incidence of vomiting as a result of adherence to the GRAD system

Effect on Vomitting	Frequency	Percent	Cum
No vomitting	56	56.00	56.00
No longer experienced	21	21.00	77.00
Reduced	12	12.00	89.00
Increased	7	7.00	96.00
Same	4	4.00	100.00
Total	**100**	**100.00**	

Correlation tested

Vomiting		
GRAD	**Reduced**	**Total**
Fully	11 (39%)	28
Partially	21 (29%)	72
Total	**32 (32%)**	**100**

Though higher among the fully following group, but the difference is statistically insignificant.

Representation of the Patients who witnessed improvement in incidence of Itching as a result of adherence to the GRAD system

Effect on Itching	Frequency	Percent	Cum
No itching	48	48.00	48.00
No longer experiences	22	22.00	70.00
Reduced	12	12.00	82.00
Same	11	11.00	93.00
Increased	7	7.00	100.00
Total	**100**	**100.00**	

Correlation tested

	Itching	
GRAD	**Improvement**	**Total**
Fully	10 (36%)	28
Partially	14 (19%)	72
Total	**34 (34%)**	**100**

Fully following group shows statistically higher improvement in itching.

Representation of the Patients who witnessed improvement in incidence of delirium as a result of adherence to the GRAD system

Effect on Delirium	Frequency	Percent	Cum
No problem	76	76.00	76.00
Increased	7	7.00	83.00
Same	7	7.00	90.00
No longer experienced	6	6.00	96.00
Reduced	4	4.00	100.00
Total	**100**	**100.00**	

Correlation tested

Delirium		
GRAD	**Reduced**	**Total**
Fully	1 (4%)	28
Partially	9 (1%)	72
Total	**10 (10%)**	**100**

Fully following group shows higher improvement in delirium.

Representation of the Patients who witnessed improvement in incidence and frequency of seizures as a result of adherence to the GRAD system

Effect on Seizures	Frequency	Percent	Cum
No seizures	92	92.00	92.00
No longer experiencing	5	5.00	97.00
Still continuing	2	2.00	99.00
Deteriorated	1	1.00	100.00
Total	**100**	**100.00**	

Correlation tested

Seizures		
GRAD	**Reduced**	**Total**
Fully	2 (7%)	28
Partially	3 (4%)	72
Total	**5 (5%)**	**100**

Fully following group shows higher improvement in seizures.

Representation of the Patients who witnessed improvement in their financial conditions as a result of adherence to the GRAD system

Change in Expenditure	Frequency	Percent
Reduced	65	65
Constant Expenditure	27	27
Paid by govt. / insurance	8	8
Total	**100**	**100**

Most of the subjects following the GRAD experienced a marked decrease in their expenditure on treatments, Dialysis and related medications and hospital visits etc.

The total expenditure incurred by the 100 subjects was reduced by enormous amount of rupees 15,47,455 per month. The average expenditure thus reduced on an average by 23,807 per person over a month for the 65 subjects who experienced a decline in their monthly expenditure.

If the subjects will recommend the GRAD system

Will they recommend	Frequency	Percent	Cum.
Yes	100	100.00	100.00
No	0	0.00	100.00
Total	**100**	**100.00**	

Results

100 dialysis patients were successfully followed between August 2021 and March 2022 and were grouped as:

Group I (who followed GRAD System fully) = 28%

Group II (who followed GRAD System partially) = 72%

53 patients were disqualified as they either failed to provide data on regular basis or could not qualify in either group.

GROUP-1 Total Patient: 28

Dialysis Status	
Dialysis Free	21
Partially Dialysis Free	7

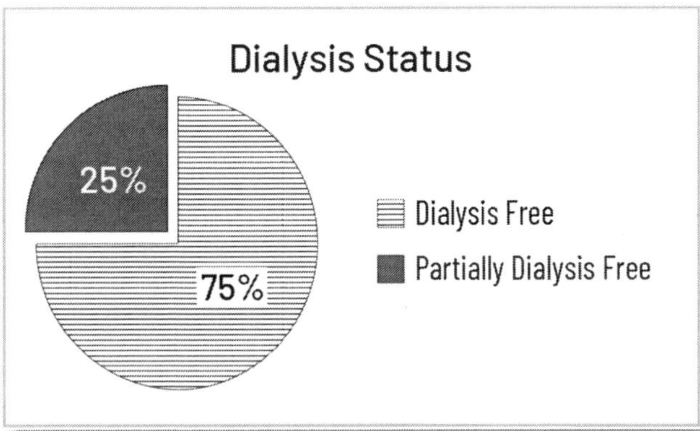

Dependence on Drugs	
Totally Drugs Free	10
Partially Drugs Free	15
No Change In Drugs	3

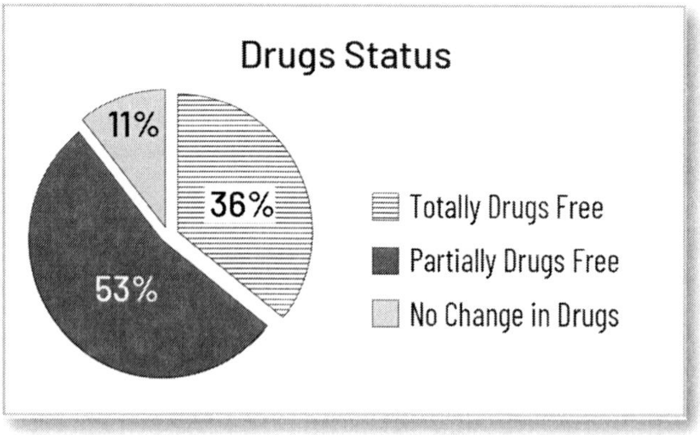

Symptomatic Relief (Vomiting/Breathlessness/Itching/Weakness/Swelling)	
More than 90% Relief	17
50% to 89% Relief	8
Relief Less than 50%	3
No Relief	0

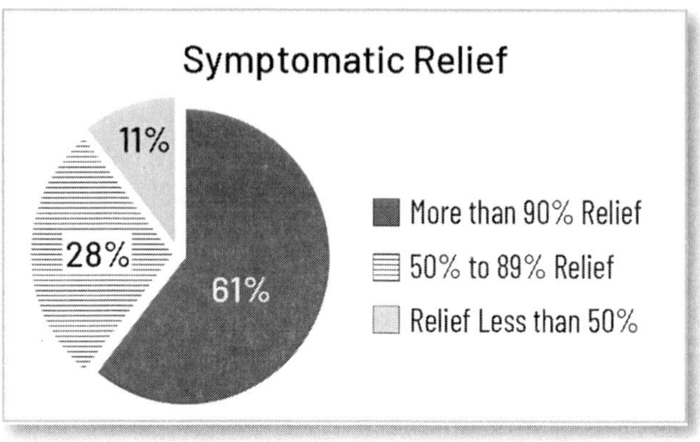

Recommending GRAD System to Others	
I will recommend to others	28
I will not recommend to others	0

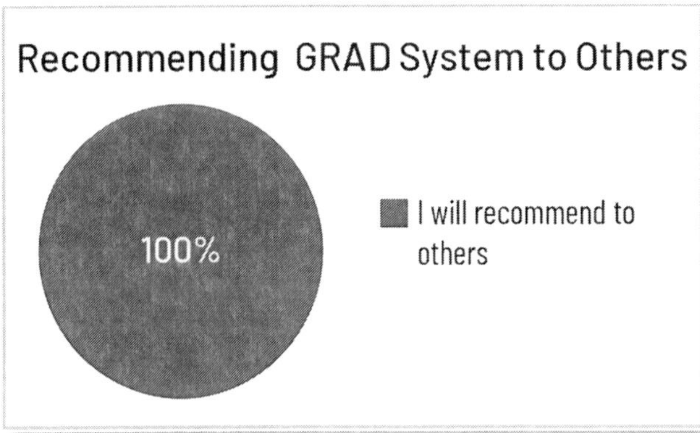

Reduction in Financial Burden	
Financial Burden Reduced to 70-90%	21
Financial Burden Reduced below 70%	7
No Reduction in Financial Burden	0

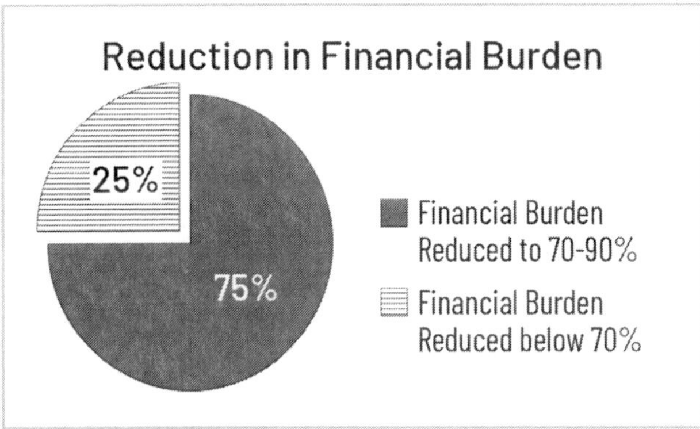

GROUP-2 Total Patient: 72

Dialysis Status	
Reduced Dialysis Frequency	42
No change in Dialysis Frequency	28
Ambiguous	2

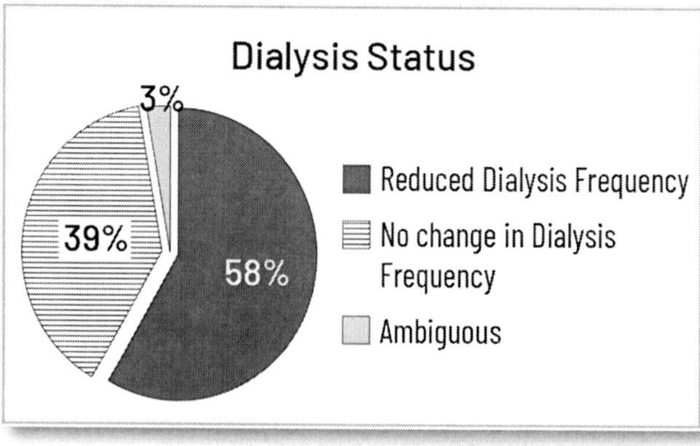

Dependence on Drugs	
Totally Drugs Free	11
Partially Drugs Free	27
No Change In Drugs	34

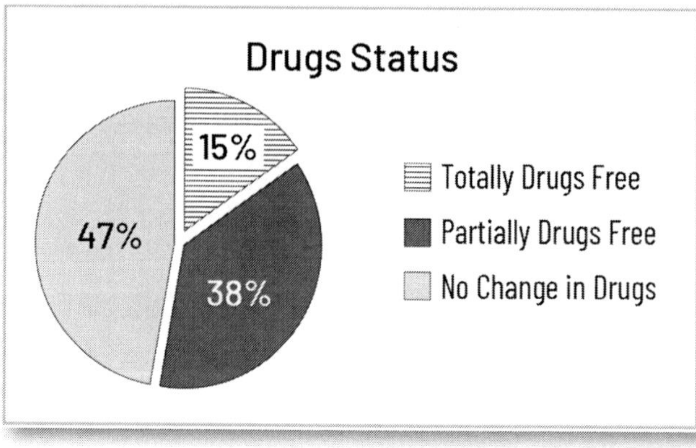

Symptomatic Relief (Vomiting/Breathlessness/Itching/Weakness/Swelling)	
More than 90% Relief	33
50 to 89% Relief	12
Relief Less than 50%	11
No Relief	2
Worse	14

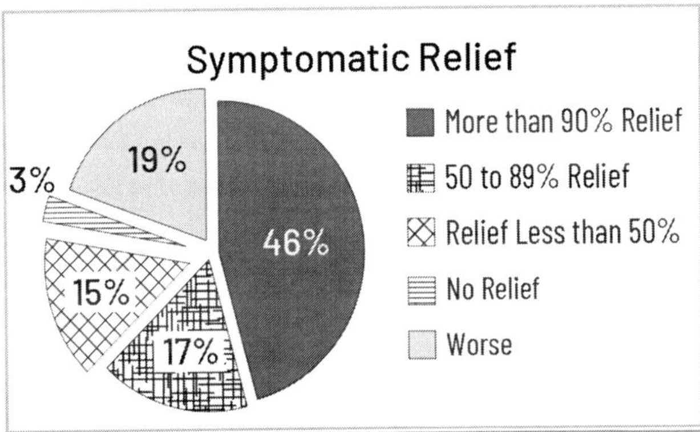

Recommend GRAD System to Other	
I will recommend to others	72
I will not recommend to others	0

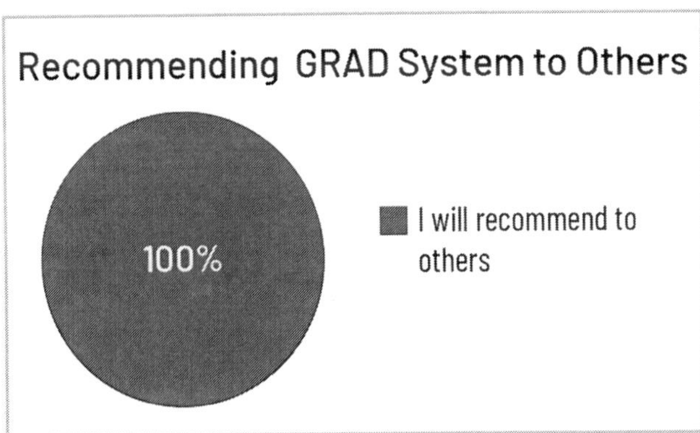

Reduction in Financial Burden	
Financial Burden Reduced to 70-90%	20
Financial Burden Reduced below 70%	17
No Reduction in Financial Burden	27
Paid by Govt. / Insurance	8

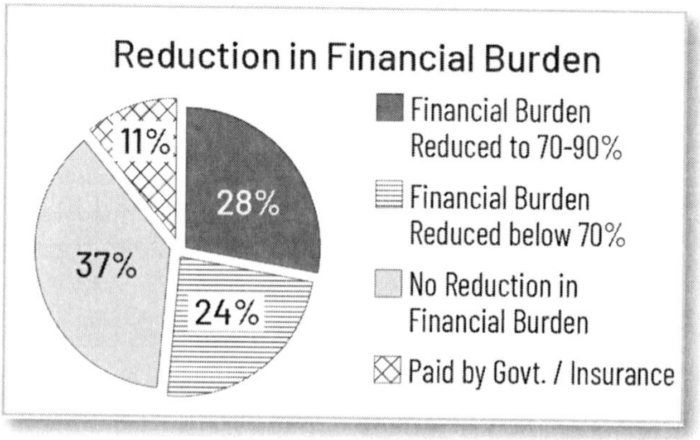

Discussion

This is a pioneering study aimed at assessing the benefits of GRAD system in reversing CKD among dialysis patients. GRAD system is an unusual amalgamation of the knowledge of human physical engineering in terms of application of gravitational force and hydrostatic pressure on human body and the principles of modern medical science for finding a cure for CKD patients. There is also an Ayurvedic angle to the system which has been derived from the thousands of years of Ayurvedic studies and deep knowledge that is recorded in ancient Indian treatises and which has been verified and found to be accurate and reliable after the employment of modern methods of verification.

Dr. Biswaroop Roy Chowdhury, the developer of the GRAD system has an impressive, wide ranging and comprehensive academic background which has enabled him to draw upon various disciplines, sciences and subjects to offer a potent combination of therapies and treatments for CKD reversal, among other pioneering breakthroughs in medical practice and theory.

In addition to being an engineering graduate and post-graduate specializing in Diabetes, he has also successfully acquired a PhD in Diabetes care. The rich diversity and innate depth in his education has helped him in combining **Physics** of the surroundings with **Chemistry** of the human body and **Biology** of the innate bodily ecosystem in human beings to reactivate, energise and resuscitate even a dying kidney. As evident from the data, CKD patients could successfully lower the burden of the disease partially/fully. Surely, GRAD system is having the potential to revolutionize the way lifestyle illnesses are treated.

GRAD system can be followed safely and with minimum resources in the privacy, security and convenience of the patient's home even in rural areas, without requiring elaborate equipment or expensive medications.

It is also seen only 28% of the patients could follow the GRAD System fully and hence, majority of the patients could not get the expected full benefit of the GRAD System. Therefore, there is a pressing need to create a GRAD System friendly environment, reliable medical ecosystem and viable infrastructure around the patients so as to make the process of following the HWI / HDT and D.I.P. Diet convenient and enjoyable. The innovative mind of the patients and their strong belief in the GRAD System is evidenced by their inventive home-based GRAD Dialysis tub. This aspect is very encouraging and relevant in regard to the wide spread and dissemination of the GRAD system and in increasing its application and effectiveness across the globe. A few of the innovative ideas are captured in the pictures given below.

INNOVATION BY PATIENTS

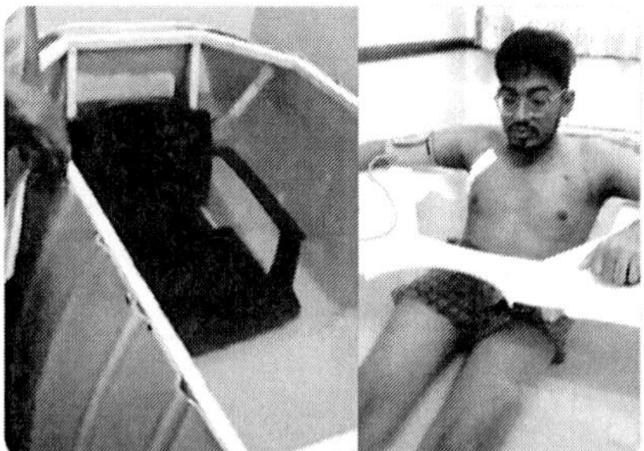

HWI with Sintex Tank

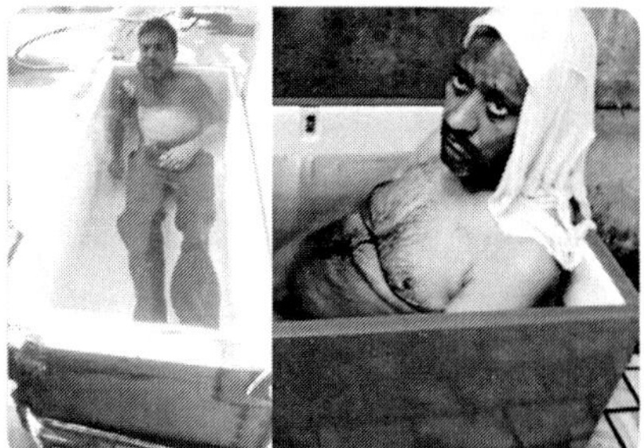

HWI with Discarded Refrigerator Body

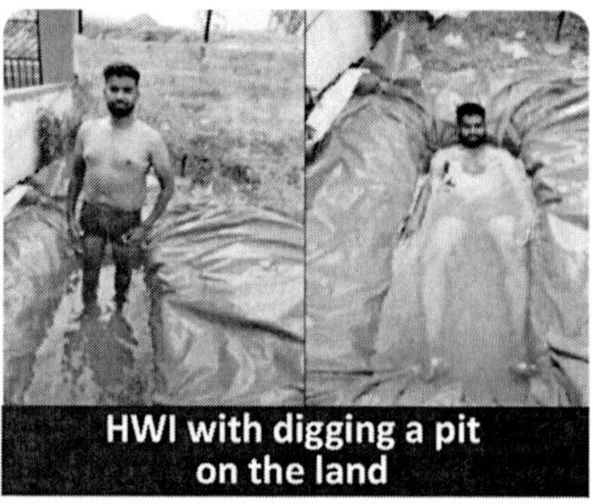

HWI with digging a pit on the land

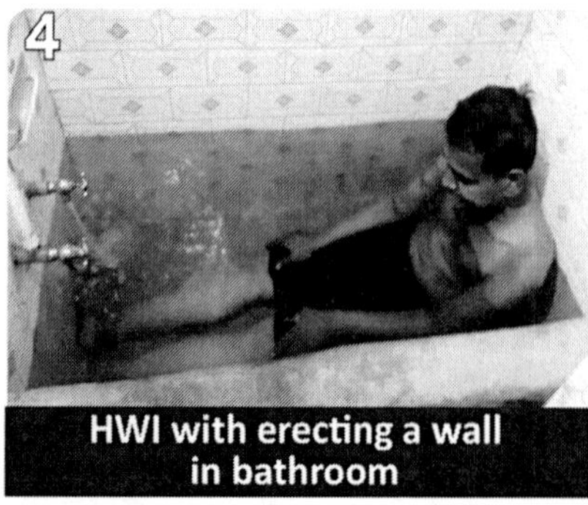

HWI with erecting a wall in bathroom

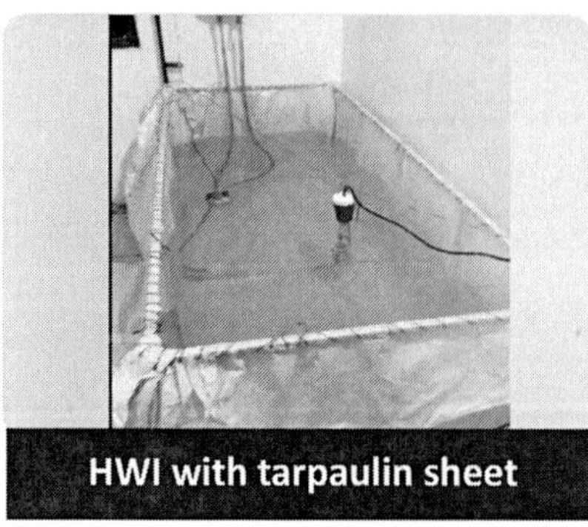

HWI with tarpaulin sheet

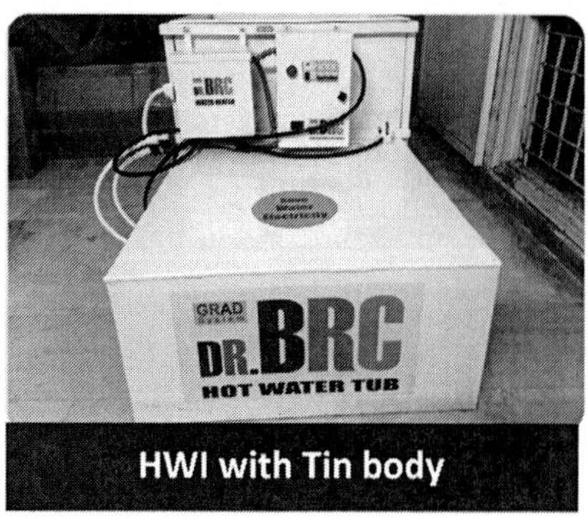

HWI with Tin body

INNOVATION BY PATIENTS

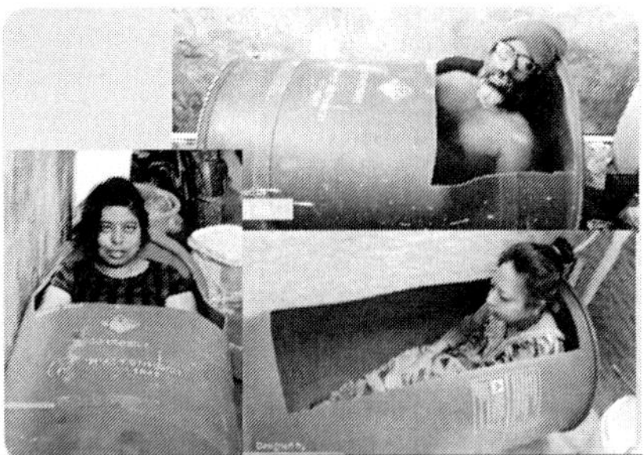

HWI with Drum

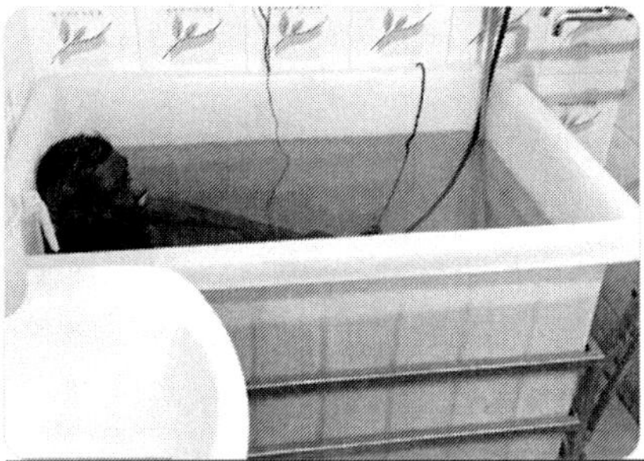

HWI with Industrial Plastic Container

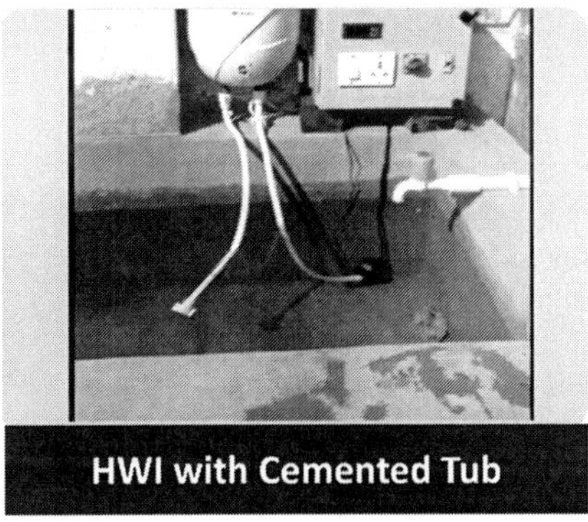

HWI with Cemented Tub

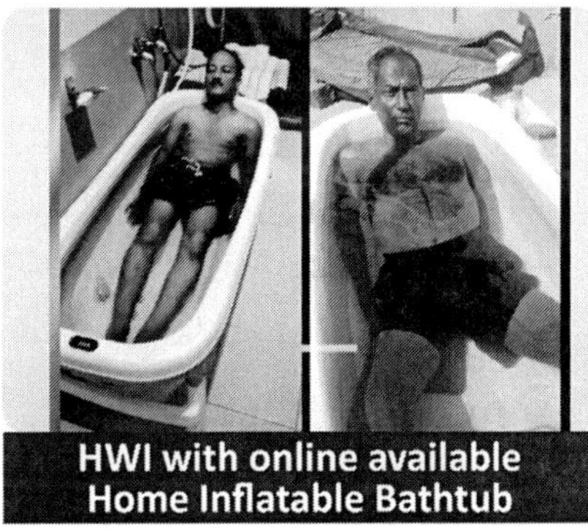

HWI with online available Home Inflatable Bathtub

90% of the patients reported a great amount of resistance and non-cooperation from their dialysis centers when the patients were in the process of reducing the frequency of dialysis in response to the improvement in their symptoms. This unfortunate, but understandable resistance from the dialysis centers (as they were losing a great deal of financial gain and patients) was a major factor why over 1/3rd of the patients discontinued the GRAD System midway. To address this issue, training, awareness and orientation programs for the medical and support staff, caretakers, patients and technicians must be regularly undertaken to teach the proper application and resultant benefit of the GRAD system all across the country.

Conclusion

GRAD system can be recommended as an effective method to reverse CKD among mild, moderate and severe CKD patients and can be seen as an effective alternative to dialysis and kidney transplant. It must be noted that no side effects or adverse events were reported during the entire study.

Scope of Further Research

✓ Impact of hot tubs on the prevalence of kidney disease in western nations where hot tubs are a part of the daily bathing rituals.... comparative analysis with nations like India where bath tubs are not in use. Has the unconscious incorporation of the hot tub treatment helped the European nations where bath tubs are frequently in use to bring down the risk of CKD.

✓ Currently, the therapy being used does not include the addition of oils, vata, pitta and grita substances as recommended in the actual Avagaha Sweda process. Further research can be conducted upon the addition of various substances to the HWI and the subsequent impact on the success of the GRAD systems.

✓ It is further suggested that Avagaha Sweda can be incorporated into modern spa culture and this would add to the efficacy of various spa treatments and boost their health giving properties and medicinal value. This treatment can prove to be highly relaxing and therapeutic for the body.

✓ It was further observed that patients on the GRAD System could reverse various comorbid conditions including diabetes and heart disease. Further study in this direction is highly recommended.

Acknowledgement

We thank all the staff who recruited and managed the study participants: Kalpana Bourai, Pratiksha Vats, Dr. Sanju Khari, Shweta Jalhotra, Ashutosh Nikhil & Rachna Sharma. We are grateful to all study participants for voluntary consent.

References

1. Clinical Trial on DIP Diet: CTRI Number CTRI/2018/12/016654 (http://ctri.nic.in/Clinicaltrials/pmaindet2.php?trialid=29268&E
2. Book: 360 Postural Medicine ISBN 978-93-5486-551-0
3. Carney, E.F. The impact of chronic kidney disease on global health. Nat Rev Nephrol 16, 251 (2020). https://doi.org/10.1038/s41581-020-0268-7
4. *Mutraghat References:*
   - Chakrapanidatta, 2008, Charaka Samhita commentary vol 1, eds Vd. Y.G. Joshi, 3rd edi., Vaidyamitra Prakashan, Pune
   - Dalhana, 1994, Sushrut Samhita Commentary, eds Yadavaji Trikamji Acharya, Chaukhamba Surbharati Prakashana, Varanasi
   - Vagbhata, 2012, Ashatangahrudaya, eds Pd. Harishashtri Paradkar, Chaukhamba Sanskrit Samsthana, Varanasi
   - Monier, Williams M.A., 2007, A Sanskrit English Dictionary, Bhartiya Granth Niketan, New Delhi
   - Agnivesh, 2013 Charak Samhita Vol 2, eds Bramhanand Tripathi, Chaukhamba Surbharati Prakashan, Varanasi
   - Sushrut, 2010, Sushrut samhita Vol 3, eds K.R. Shreekanth Murthy, Chaukhamba Orientalia, Varanasi
   - Sushrut, 2017, Sushrut samhita Vol.1, eds K.R. Shreekanth Murthy, Chaukhamba Orientalia, Varanasi
   - Ambikadatta shashtri, 2008, Bhaishajyaratnavali, Chaukhamba Prakashan, Varanasi, 19th edition
   - Mahanta Rabi Narayan, Panda P.K., 2014, A Patho-clinical study on the disorders of Mutrabaha Strotas with its Modern Interpretation W.S.R. to Mutraghata, International Journal of Herbal Medicine 2014:1(5):33-41

5. Global Dialysis Perspective: India, Joyita Bharati and Vivekanand Jha KIDNEY360 1: 1143–1147, 2020. doi: https://doi.org/10.34067/KID.0003982020 (Bharati and Jha, 2020).
6. International Society of Nephrology (ISN): https://www.theisn.org/blog/2020/11/27/more-than-850-million-worldwide-have-some-form-of-kidney-disease-help-raise-awareness/
7. Volicer L, Jean-Charles R, Chobani an AV. Effects of head-down tilt on fluid and electrolyte balance. Aviation Space Environ Med. 1976 Oct;47(10):1065-8. PMID: 985278.5.
8. *References for Awgaha Sweda*
    - Charak Samhita / sutra sthan / chapter 14
    - https://www.koreascience.or.kr/article/JAKO201925454134689.pdf
9. Cardiovascular & Renal Effects of Head-Out Water immersion in Man. Circulation Research Vol 39, No. 5, Nov 1976
10. Immersion in thermoneutral water: Effects on atrial compliance. December 2006, Aviation Space and Environmental AMedicine 77(11):1183-7
11. Acute and chronic effects of hot water immersion on inflammation and metabolism in sedentary overweight adults. J Appl. Physiol 125:2008-2018
12. Effects of water immersion on renal function in the nephrotic syndrome. Kidney International Vol 21 (1982), PP.395-401
13. Reversal of Type 1 Diabetes Using Plant Based Diet: A Case Study. Journal of the Science of Healing Outcomes ISSN 2347-8438
14. *Reference:*
    - Sushruta Samhita, Nibandhasamgraha commentary of Dalhana,
    - Nyayachandrika commentary of Gayadasa, edited by Yadavji Trikamjee Acharya and Narayan Ram Acharya, Chaukhamba Orientalia, Varanasi, Reprint, 2009; 386
15. *Reference*:
    - Charaka Samhita Siddisthana–9 (Trimarmiya Siddhi adhyaya)
    - Ashtanga Hridaya Samhita Nidanasthana–9 (Mutraghata Nidana adhyaya)
    - Ashtanga Hridaya Samhita Chiktsasthana–1 1 (Mutraghata Chikitsa adhyaya
    - Madavanidana–3 1 (Mutraghata Nidana adhyaya)

16. Su. Utt. 58/17; Ch .Si. 9/34; A.H.Ni.9/37
17. Da.Su.Utt.58/17
18. Gianfaldoni S, Tchernev G, Wollina U, et al. History of the Baths and Thermal Medicine. Open Access Maced J Med Sci. 2017; 5(4):566-568. Published 2017 Jul 23. doi:10.3889/oamjms.2017.126
19. van Tubergen A, van der Linden S *A brief history of spa therapy-Annals of the Rheumatic Diseases* 2002; 61:273-275

Section - II

FAQs

Frequently Asked Questions and Important Instructions for CKD Patients

Question: How important is Creatinine level for CKD / Dialysis patients? What is the scientific base of it?

Answer: High Creatinine is Not Your Enemy!

Creatinine is a word that you must have heard, mostly in relation to its increase in the body of Kidney patients. It is a scary and dangerous word that is accepted by one and all if Creatinine levels increase in the body. Let us understand what does it mean to have an increased level of Creatinine and all of your fears related to this word will vanish. And as soon as the fear related to creatinine levels vanishes, all the kidney patients in our country will at least reduce by half. This is because they will cease to be kidney patients.

Ask your doctor what is the normal level of Creatinine in the body and he will tell you that it is up to 1.2 mg per decilitre. Then ask, what if the Creatinine levels increase beyond this normal figure? He will respond that your kidneys are not functioning well and you are unwell. You then ask him a question clearly about how much of an increase in the Creatinine levels in the human body can result in his or her death? Will the individual die if the Creatinine levels increase by a 100% or even by a 1000%? The answer is 'No'. Now if the Creatinine level increases by over 2000%, say, 24 mg per decilitre? If Creatinine is dangerous then there must be a threshold beyond which an individual must be closer to a dangerous level and he or she may die. What is that threshold?

You will be surprised to know that there is no such threshold in the human body. When they say that Creatinine is the body's waste, it is not mandatory that it really is the body's waste. Creatinine is not your enemy. It has a lot of functions. Instead, its opposite holds true in case of death. Those individuals with lower-than-normal Creatinine levels die earlier as compared to those whose Creatinine levels are higher than normal.

The world's largest trial which was a study conducted amongst 5,388 kidney patients and continued for several years. It was noted that the patients with lower-than-normal Creatinine levels died earlier as compared to those patients who had higher than normal Creatinine levels in their body. Try to understand this. There is no such correlation that if your Creatinine levels are low then your kidney is healthy and if your Creatinine levels are high then your kidney is unhealthy. The opposite, however, is true and is backed by evidence.

Creatinine levels increase when the body has more muscles. More the muscles break down in the body more will be the creation of Creatinine levels. If an individual has fewer muscles, his support structure is not good and is fragile in nature. So, they have a tendency to die earlier.

More Creatinine levels in the body are indicative of the individual having more muscles in his body. Alternatively, if you exercise more often and build muscles, the Creatinine levels in the body will subsequently increase. This has no relation with the proper or improper functioning of the kidney.

Secondly, in case you have a bacterial infection, then there is a tendency for the Creatinine levels to increase in your body. This is because Creatinine fights the bacterial infection in the body like our immunity.

Thirdly, when you take in large quantities of steroids, if you take medicines like Aspirin on a regular basis, then your Creatinine levels will increase in the body. This is a protective mechanism of the body such that the steroid's damage in the body can be controlled. Here too, there is no connection between the increased Creatinine levels and malfunctioning of the kidneys.

Fourthly, you can conduct an experiment by yourself. Get your Creatinine levels checked to begin with. Then after the test, all those who consume non-vegetarian food, must eat stomach full of non-vegetarian food, especially red meat. After two hours get your Creatinine levels checked again. The results will show an increase by 3-4 times. This is because when you eat animal food, you literally eat Creatinine which is then absorbed into the blood stream from the stomach. This will result in an increase in the Creatinine level in the blood. Does this entail that the kidney is unhealthy because of increased Creatinine levels in the body?

Finally, if your kidney is not functioning properly and is unable to flush out the toxins then it may result in an increase in the Creatinine levels in the body. It is merely one of the five factors responsible for increase in Creatinine levels in the body.

So if anybody's Creatinine levels increase in the body, it can be because of any of the five factors just discussed. Out of these four reasons are positive in nature and only one is negative. But it has been observed that when a patient visits a doctor with increased levels of Creatinine, then the doctors immediately conclude that the patient is a Kidney failure patient.

All that is needed to prove that you have high levels of Creatinine in your body is to feed you a cooked meal of red meat. When you eat animal food including dairy products, you are eating Creatinine.

On the one hand we say Creatinine is waste and on the other hand that is what we consume in form of animal food. Moreover, when the Creatinine level increases in the body, we blame it on the Kidneys. So if the Creatinine levels increase in your body you tend to conclude that your kidneys are malfunctioning. This is a muddled diagnostic conclusion.

Take a simple example where one has to identify injured people from non-injured ones using binoculars. It's quite simple, all you have to do is look for the visible blood spots on their body. Those who have more blood on their body are badly injured while the ones with less blood or no blood are less injured or not injured at all.

Here the point to understand is that every red spot might not be blood. There could be some spill of juice or tomato sauce or something red.

Here we can conclude that every red spot is considered blood even if it is some red juice or tomato sauce or red color and any person with a red spot is identified as an injured person even if he is not! The same way high Creatinine level of every patient is considered as a case of kidney failure even if he is not!

As a part of a conspiracy, they make you believe that your kidney is malfunctioning. The next step is to make you take up a dialysis session. It is worth mentioning here, that once the body undergoes Dialysis, the kidney thinks that all its work is being done externally and gradually starts shutting down. This results in the decrease in urine output than before and consequently, he truly becomes a dialysis dependent kidney patient. This means that kidney patients are being manufactured as against being naturally so.

First, they will prove that your Creatinine levels are high and then make you undergo one Dialysis procedure and that is enough to convert a healthy individual into a kidney patient. Now his urine output is not normal and the individual will keep needing dialysis on a recurring basis thereafter.

It is worth mentioning that dialysis is a One lakh crore worth business. It is unfortunate that dialysis patients spend about INR 50,000 per month on treatment. The patient also has an attendant who accompanies him on a full-time basis, often leaving his job to take care of the ailing patient. So, it can be said that among all the available diseases the most painful disease is that of a patient of Dialysis.

Question: Should a CKD patient worry about Potassium as during therapies several reports indicate an increase in Potassium levels in the patient.

Answer: The Potassium measured in blood is the extracellular Potassium. However, the problem in the body is caused by intracellular Potassium which we don't measure. When we do not take in animal proteins, the intracellular potassium doesn't lock as much in the cell. On the contrary, when animal proteins are taken, then this intracellular potassium gets locked in the cells. Therefore, Potassium and Potassium rich foods must not be a cause of worry. By animal proteins it is meant non-vegetarian food, milk and milk products like paneer, cheese, butter, ghee, curd etc.

Question: What about the fruits and vegetables high in Potassium?

Answer: Before starting the GRAD protocol for treatment, patients must unlearn certain things. The treatment and diet advised is being conducted very scientifically and must not be a cause to worry. We must understand that what you eat does not directly get thrown into your blood. Food first reaches the gut, which is also known as the second brain, as it can process and filter the waste out and let the needed amount of nutrient travel into the blood. However the gut can do its function best if you eat plant based food in its natural / raw state.

Question: What is the connection between fistula and high BP in a CKD patient?

Answer: The human body's natural tendency to expel a foreign element is by raising its Blood Pressure. So, if a fistula is attached to the body, then according to the new standard for a kidney failure patient, the Blood Pressure will be more than normal. When the patient's relatives and friends discuss this increase in the Blood Pressure, s/he gets agitated resulting in a further increase in the BP. It is therefore, advised to the kidney failure patients not to get alarmed, when they observe their BP rising after implanting fistula.

Question: How will CKD /dialysis patients be monitored on a daily basis?

Answer: Patients are monitored through the **GRAD APP** which can be downloaded from **Google Playstore.** Please go through the following instructions carefully especially the Kidney or Dialysis patients who are associated with Dr. Biswaroop Roy Chowdhury through virtual OPD or through clinics or are even admitted in HIIMS Hospitals.

You have to be careful of a few things to get freedom from Dialysis and Kidney disease. You have to be in consonance with Dr. Biswaroop's doctors and paramedic staff.

On a daily basis you must share PRAN data and this data should be shared through the App namely **"GRAD APP Patient"** available on play store.

Now let us understand which data is required from the patients by the paramedics that will help them decide if there is any improvement in their kidneys and if there is a need for further dialysis for the treatment.

Alternatively, it will help to decide if your therapy needs to be changed to suit your health condition or even change the duration of the Head Down Tilt therapy or the Hot Water Immersion Therapy. The data shared will help the doctors/paramedics evaluate if the temperature for the treatment or the angle of tilt needs to be altered or not. There are several such decisions that they need to take towards the treatment of a dialysis patient for which they need certain data on a regular basis.

So, wherever you are undergoing the treatment (through GRAD system) for kidney disease, be it at home, or at the hospital, or even at the clinics, your data must reach them on a daily basis.

The first data that is needed from Day 1 of the treatment is that of the Blood Pressure (BP). The BP must be monitored before and after undergoing the Head Down Tilt Therapy. The BP after the therapy is expected to be lesser.

Similarly, you must monitor the BP both before and after undergoing the Hot Water Immersion Treatment.

So it can be said that for both the therapies you would be monitoring four readings each. In addition to this, they would be requiring your weight before and after the Hot Water Immersion therapy.

Remember to get out of water, dry yourself completely, and only then measure your weight. It has been observed that after the Hot Water Immersion Therapy, the patient's weight reduces from 200 grams up to 1 Kg or even more. This weight is nothing but the fluid that has been released by the body in form of perspiration which is a very good thing.

In addition, in case you have swelling in your body, you need to record if the swelling reduced after either of the two therapies.

One of the very important and critical data that is required from the patients is that of Urine output. Those patients whose urine output is below 400ml must measure their urine output as accurately as possible. So every time you urinate, do so in a measuring cup. You get these measuring cups in varying capacities so you can choose one according to your comfort level. So ultimately, you need to measure the total urine output in 24 hours and mention it in the GRAD App.

Finally, all the symptoms you experience throughout the day, be it weakness, itching, head ache, vomiting, diarrhoea, etc. Whatever be the factors that trigger discomfort as a result of the therapies, must be mentioned in the GRAD APP.

On the basis of these figures and explanations of a patient's day, doctors/ paramedics decide the course of action for him or her for the next day in the form of 'recommendation' through the GRAD APP. This includes the diet, the degree of tilt of therapy or the heat in the hot water etc. Also through your data which is everyday shared through GRAD APP, doctors/paramedics will be able to decide whether you need the dialysis next day or not.

It becomes easier to take the right and appropriate decisions for the benefit of the patient based on the data provided by the patient through GRAD APP.

It is therefore, expected that each patient will diligently co-operate by sharing accurate data on a daily basis, wherever you may be situated. This data sheet will be the basis for your treatment to take the correct and appropriate course.

You must also make an effort to understand why are these therapies recommended for you, why is the diet chosen to be so for you, how will the kidney revive once it has failed functioning, how can the dialysis stop for you etc. Towards this, you must endeavour to understand the science of bodily function as this will help you experience benefits of the treatment in a clearer manner. **For this, you can read the book available on the hyperlink, www.biswaroop.com/360degree.**

The book, **'360° Postural Medicine'** is available in form of an eBook in both Hindi as well as English.

You can also request for the physical book from your doctor if you are in the HIIMS hospital. In case you are virtual OPD patient, you will be couriered the book in either Hindi or English, as requested by you.

In other words, you need to educate yourself so that you will be able to comprehend why is this specific therapy applicable on you and how will it benefit you. How will the therapy help in stopping the dialysis or avoiding the transplant for good? How can Kidney failure be reversed through this therapy?

You will also be able to learn from the book that if you suffer from other ailments along with kidney failure, like Diabetes etc., how will you be able to cure them rapidly as well?

The more awareness you generate and more knowledge you acquire around it, the more beneficial it will be for you. For this you need to share accurate daily data through GRAD APP with your doctors. Hopefully with this methodology you will very quickly be able to be dialysis-free and reverse your kidney issues completely.

Question: While following the GRAD system, what are the symptoms or conditions in which we have to take the patient for Emergency Dialysis?
Answer: The following below mentioned symptoms and their parameters will warn you and indicate that you should take the patient for Emergency Dialysis.

Vomiting / itching / excessive swelling / breathlessness / delirium / extreme weakness / negligible urine output / daily weight gain more than 300 gm/day.

Question: While doing HWI or HDT if breathlessness issue arises, then what step should we take?

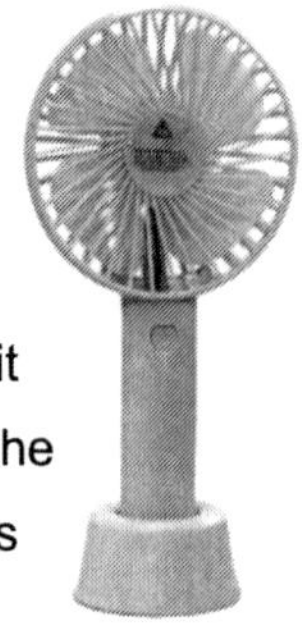

Answer: Take a hand held (battery operated) fan and keep it in front of your face and take deep breaths. Discontinue therapy if breathlessness persists. That means you have to do HWI and HDT only for the time period till you can do it comfortably without breathlessness. Then slowly increase the time as your body adjusts and doesn't face breathlessness any more.

Question: What to do in case we feel weakness while doing HWI or HDT

Answer: a) Wrap wet towel around head.

b) Do the therapy till you feel comfortable. As soon as weakness or fatigue is felt discontinue the therapy. Then gradually increase the time of HWI and HDT as per comfort and convenience of the body without facing any weakness. It is recommended that the first day instead of sitting for 2 hr. session of HDT and HWI each, patients should start with half an hour of HWI and HDT to familiarize the body with the therapies and then gradually increase the time according to comfort level or symptomatic discomforts. As soon as discomforts start, discontinue the therapy. To complete the 2 hrs session you can take the therapy in installments – half an hour each for four sessions or one hour each in 2 sessions.

Question: What results may the patients get if they pursue HWI and HDT only for one hour daily instead of two hours daily?

Answer: They won't get 100% results; they will get partial results. However, most of the patients are not able to do the therapies for 2 hrs. each due to symptomatic discomforts such as breathlessness or weakness. In this case, as explained above they should start their therapies in installments and gradually increase their time to 2 hrs. as their body feels comfortable without facing any symptomatic discomforts. This is more like a hit and trial method. A patient will need to understand his own body and within the comforts of his body he can carry on and implement those rules in his lifestyle.

Question: How to taper down the drugs while doing HWI or HDT or while following the GRAD System?

Answer: The most important thing to understand here is that while following the GRAD System, blood pressure and blood sugar (if you are on blood sugar medicine) will start getting normalized very fast. So, every day you have to check your Blood Pressure and Blood sugar and accordingly with the help of your physician you have to taper down your medicine. Even medication for thyroid etc. need to be tapered as your thyroid levels also normalize. For this you have to keep on doing thyroid test every month and based on your improvement, refer to your physician for tapering your thyroid medicine. All kinds of supplements must be stopped. If you are on heart related medicine, it may need to be readjusted, for which refer to your doctor.

Question: How to know if I have to go for dialysis or not and if I have to go for dialysis, what is the right time?

Answer: As far as possible, the consideration must be symptomatic. If there are no symptoms then as much as possible the patient must avoid dialysis. For the benefit of the patients who are under supervision through Virtual OPD or HIIMS, they are expected to fill their parameters on daily basis through GRAD APP. Based on their entries, our experts (doctors/ paramedics) recommend whether they need to go for dialysis or not.

Question: I have been on GRAD system and Diet Protocol but did not get any benefit out of it or my dialysis frequency did not decrease?

Answer: The answer to your question is the Prospective Cohort Study in section I. Please read that carefully. Once you will read that you will understand that you have not followed protocol as per the GRAD system fully. You will realize that you have either been doing some mistake while doing the HWI and HDT Therapy or not following the appropriate diet. It is proven through the study that 98% of the patients are benefitted by avoiding transplant or stopped dialysis or supporting drugs, decreased frequency of dialysis, or reduced dependency on supporting drugs within 100 days of following the GRAD Protocol. Only in very rare 2% of the cases because of unknown factors it may take longer than 100 days to heal or reverse CKD.

Question: Once we start GRAD system, in how many days will we get cured?

Answer: Again, read the prospective cohort study given in section-1. You will see that many of the patients could free themselves of the dialysis and supporting drugs within a span of 100 days. On the other hand some of the patients did not get much relief but may take more time to reverse their disease. This means most of the patients get full or partial benefit within 100 days. Only few rarest of the rare cases may not be able to heal themselves due to unknown causes.

We strongly recommend that you try the GRAD System for one week. If you see any light of improvement in any of the aspects, then you can take a decision to continue for another week. In case you do not see any improvement in any of the parameters or observe worsening of symptoms, you may take the decision to discontinue the GRAD System.

Question: What do you suggest for those who fall in the rarest of the rare 2% cases who could not benefit from the GRAD system or GRAD system is not suitable for them?

Answer: It may be noted that due to the diet and lifestyle modification recommended in GRAD system, the first positive signs are seen within 1 week to 10 days' time. First 7 to 10 days are quite critical. After 7 days you have to ask yourself if you have observed any improvement in your health condition. If yes, you can decide to continue the diet. However, in 7-10 days' time if you see no improvement or observe worsening of symptoms, you can discontinue the diet and lifestyle modification and go back to your original system. Do not forget to report to us regarding no improvement or worsening of condition.

Question: Are there any safety precaution to be followed while doing HDT/HWI?

Answer: If you are a patient suffering from Kidney Failure and are undergoing treatment through our **Gravitational Resistance and Diet (GRAD) System**, then you must ensure certain safety tips. These safety measures must be followed without fail when you undergo the **Hot Water Therapy (HWT) and the Head Down Tilt (HDT) Therapy.**

The 6 S of Safety Measures

Slowly

When undergoing HDT or HWI therapies, it is not necessary that the patient starts with two hours of treatment on the first day itself. It is advisable to start slowly and then gradually increase the treatment duration as per the comfort and stamina of the body.

For example, on Day 1 of the treatment one can start with 30 minutes of HWI / HDT therapy. As soon as the body gives out signals of uneasiness or discomfiture, s/he can stop the treatment for the day. The symptoms vary from mild dizziness, vomiting, uneasiness, unable to bear the heat or tilt of the body etc. As soon as these symptoms start, the patient can take a break from the session or end that session.

It is important to remember that during the Hot Water Immersion Therapy, although the patient merely sits in water, the pressure on the body above the water is lesser than the pressure under water. This pressure difference combined with the heat of 40°C results in certain changes in the body which can be compared to the changes a body undergoes by being regular at the gymnasium.

So, despite being in a static position, the patient's body undergoes a lot of changes. Therefore, it is evident that despite sitting in hot water for only a short duration, the patient might experience tiredness or even exhaustion which is without doubt a positive change. Nonetheless, the patient must observe caution and start the treatment slowly and gradually increase the therapy time duration only when s/he feels comfortable in doing so.

Similarly, in the Head Down Tilt Therapy, it has been observed that around 10% of the patients experience mild head-aches after 10-20 minutes of tilting the head. As soon as the patients experience this sort of discomfiture, it is advisable for them to discontinue the therapy session. It must not be considered that these symptoms are signaling danger. Merely because of a change of posture, the body uses Gravitational pull towards its benefit to achieve a certain goal. This is the reason why initially the body might experience minor discomfort as it aligns itself to the new angle.

This can be understood through an example. If someone who is not used to running long distances suddenly starts running, s/he is likely to experience a kind of pain resulting from the muscle pull in the legs. This pain is indicative of the fact that the individual's muscles had been inactive for a long time. When these muscles were suddenly put to use by running, the body underwent a few changes, resulting in an experience of pain or discomfiture.

This pain in legs does not point towards any sort of danger, but we can surely learn that it arises due to the activity in certain muscles or a certain part of the body that the body was not used to previously. In our case it can be seen in the **Head Down Tilt Therapy** as well as the **Hot Water Immersion Therapy.**

Therefore, the first point of safety is **Slowly.** It is recommended that the patients start either of the therapies with **30 to 45 minutes** of treatment only and observe the changes that the body undergoes. Let the body get accustomed to the changes slowly and only then increase the time duration of the therapy gradually.

It is worth mentioning here that there are patients who sit in hot water or a head down tilt position for two hours on the first day itself without experiencing any discomfort or pain. They experience healing and relief from pain in their kidneys from the very first day of treatment proving that each body is an individual with varying experiences.

Another way to complete one's treatment, therefore, might be to take the treatment sessions of 30 to 45 minutes two to three times a day. This way the patient will be able to complete the designated two hours of therapy without experiencing drastic changes and discomfort. It is important to start slowly, whatever be the capacity of the individual. It is not advisable to start the treatment with a single sitting of two hours despite discomfort or pain just because it has been prescribed for that patient.

Again Slowly

The second step of safety that is of crucial importance is Again Slowly, especially when the patient is coming out of the Hot Water Immersion Therapy or the Head Down Tilt Therapy. One must be careful and not get out of the therapy with a sudden jolt. It is important to remember that in the Hot Water Therapy the pressure difference on the patient's body above and below the water is of 2%. The changes that the body undergoes through the HWI treatment are because of this pressure difference. If the patient gets out of the water suddenly then the pressure difference may cause a disbalance in the body. This can either result in dizziness or the patient might even faint at times. A patient's body is already fragile, and this pressure difference can impact their health condition.

Even those individuals who are healthy and not suffering any malady, when you wake up from sleep, be careful that you don't get out of bed with a jolt. Take your time and slowly wake up and sit on the bed. Next, move your hand and feet fingers and flex your neck in all four directions and slowly stand on your feet. This is the right way to get out of bed.

When you are asleep, your blood flow is in a particular direction because of the Gravitational pull and when you suddenly sit up straight to a 90° angle, the gravitational pull gets disbalanced which may sometimes even cause a cardiac arrest.

Therefore, specifically after a Head Down Tilt Therapy or a Hot Water Immersion Therapy when you get up, make sure you are slow and careful about it. Move the fingers of your hands and feet, flex your neck in all directions, and get up with the help of your attendant to ensure you don't suffer any ill effects.

As you must have observed that the way the astronauts come down to the earth from their space ships, initially they are unable to stand up on their own and only with the help of a few people do they stand. Once their body familiarizes itself with the earth's atmosphere and environment then they are able to perform normal movement.

On the same ground when the patient's body is submerged in water, their body is able to feel a different pressure due to gravity. That is why it is critical for them to get up really slowly be it any therapy that they are undergoing or even waking up from sleep.

Check the movement of fingers, move your neck from side to side, or even roll your shoulders in clockwise and anticlockwise directions and slowly get up and out of bed.

Stomach

The third S of the safety measure stands for stomach. A patient is advised to undergo both the therapies on an **'empty stomach'**. In case one chooses to eat something before the therapies, there is a chance for acidity to build up in the system resulting in vomiting or nausea. Therefore, it is advised to undergo the Head Down Tilt Therapy first thing in the morning on an empty stomach and the Hot Water Immersion Therapy just before bedtime at night. For this there must be a minimum gap of two hours between dinner and the therapy.

Systolic Blood Pressure

This is the fourth S of the safety measures to be adopted by patients adopting the GRAD System for treatment. When undergoing both the therapies every patient must measure their blood pressure prior to the treatment. It is important to know that a patient suffering from kidney disease has a tendency to suffer from high blood pressure. So if your systolic blood pressure is above 180 then you must avoid the Head Down Tilt Therapy. This therapy is safe as long as the blood pressure is below 180. In case your blood pressure is above 180, then before attempting the Head Down Tilt Therapy, one must make efforts to bring down the blood pressure.

A simple technique that can be adopted to bring down the systolic blood pressure is the Lower Leg Hot Water Immersion Therapy. Take a bucket with hot water at 42°C and immerse both the legs in it for 20 to 30 mins. Now check your blood pressure again. If it comes down to 180 or lower, then you are free to do the Head Down Tilt Therapy.

Hot Water Immersion Therapy can be done at any blood pressure as the therapy automatically works on reducing the blood pressure of the body. On the other hand, the Head Down Tilt Therapy first works on increasing the blood pressure and finally reduces it. Both the therapies ultimately bring down the blood pressure levels in a patient.

Safety Belt

On either side of the Dialysis tub is attached a **'safety belt'**. It is recommended to all patients using the Dialysis tub to always secure themselves with the safety belt before starting the Hot Water Immersion Therapy. A patient in pain sitting in hot water might experience peace and serenity during the treatment, resulting in sleep while inside the hot water tub. This can result in the patient sliding inside the water unknowingly. In rare cases, when a patient is too fragile, s/he might faint while sitting in water and therefore, slide under the water. Alternatively, a patient who is very light weight might float in the water in the tub and in the process slip into the water.

Therefore, it is imperative for a patient to secure themselves with the safety belt to avoid mishaps during the treatment.

Standing Nearby

A patient undergoing either Hot Water Immersion Therapy or the Head Down Tilt Therapy must ensure to have someone standing nearby throughout the treatment. The attendant must also be alert and aware of the patient's health during the therapy.

For Hot Water Immersion Therapy conducted in our hospital, we use an electrical safety panel attached to the tub. This panel cuts off any electricity that might get discharged into the water. You must have noticed that when you use the geyser at home for hot water, then despite the geyser being switched on 24 hours, the current never reaches the taps or the water. All you get is hot water to use. However, it has been noticed in the rarest cases that the current has succeeded in reaching the water due to the fault of the geyser, thus, electrifying the user in varying degrees.

Being mindful of such rare instances, we have installed a safety panel that switches off the main power supply in case there is a fault in the geyser and the electrical current might reach the water. The intermediary panel works between the geyser and dialysis tub, ensuring safety for the patient undergoing the therapy.

So when a patient is undergoing the Hot Water Immersion therapy at their own premises, then it is important to have an attendant standing by. The therapy by itself is very safe and has no side effects whatsoever on the patient. Still as a precautionary measure as the patient is in a fragile health condition, it is advisable to have somebody nearby who can keep an eye during the entire treatment duration. There are several hazards that are beyond human control that are possible in any given environment. To avoid any such mishap, it is critical that the patient ensures a trustworthy, alert, and healthy attendant to keep a watchful eye all through the treatment.

These are the six safety features that each patient must ensure during both the therapy sessions. Ask yourselves if you have ensured each of these measures before the therapy and only then start with the treatment.

Question: How to handle some common issues/discomforts faced by CKD patients without the help of drugs and doctors/while sitting at home

Ascites	➢ Wrap Banana leaf over abdomen and lie in sunlight for at least 2 hours ➢ Lower Leg Hot Water Immersion (LLHWI)
Breathlessness	➢ Chew ginger ➢ Prone ventilation ➢ Deep Breathing
Urine output low	➢ Lower Leg Hot Water Immersion before going to sleep ➢ HWI up to 3 hours ➢ Cucumber juice/Radish juice 30 ml-2 times in a day ➢ Water retention/Swelling ➢ Lower Leg Hot Water Immersion before going to sleep ➢ HWI up to 3 hours ➢ Cucumber juice/Radish juice 30 ml-2 times in a day
Severe weakness after HWI	➢ Drink green juice/Red juice/lemon water during HWI
Headache after HDT	➢ Deep breathing exercise
Severe vomiting	➢ Chew one small pieces of ginger, do not eat anything after 45 minutes of vomit. Keep green. ➢ Cardamom in mouth throughout the day (when not eating anything). ➢ Have 100 ml lemon water sip wise.
Itching and rashes on the body	➢ Apply Cold pressed coconut oil mixed with a pinch of Potash alum (fitkari)
Loss of Appetite	➢ Chew fennel seeds (saunf) 3 times a day after every meal ➢ Walk 30 minutes

Weakness	➢ Make a dip of 1 inch giloy stem, 15-20 holy basil leaves, 8 to 10 soaked munnakha and 1 tsp aloe vera pulp. Mix together and make a paste, consume 2 tsp in one day in morning and evening. ➢ Have one small bowl of dry roasted Makhana (foxnut) once in a day ➢ 100 ml lemon water once in a day
High BP	➢ Lower leg Hot water immersion ➢ Banana Stem juice-40ml (If BP is >160/100)
Body ache/Pain in legs	➢ Night Jasmine decoction ➢ Massage with sesame oil warmed with 3-4 Garlic cloves
Blurred vision	➢ Sun gazing during sunrise and sunset for 15 min with break in between ➢ Wash eyes with Triphla water (after sieving)
Blood in Urine	➢ Raw diet without cooked food ➢ Fasting with green juice, Red Juice, Vegetable juice, lemon water
Blood in stool	➢ Sitz Bath ➢ Raw diet ➢ Wet Cotton Bandage
Constipation	➢ Fresh Amla juice 20 ml + 20 ml water in morning, 40 minutes before breakfast ➢ Soaked Munakkha (3-4) once in a day
Loose motions	➢ 100ml lemon water. ➢ Coconut water once in a day if Potassium level is upto 6
Cold and Cough	➢ 3 Step heat protocol

Question: Whom to call in case of emergency?

Answer: Those CKD patients who are being monitored through Virtual OPD or Post HIIMS can reach doctors/paramedics through Emergency Helpline number available 24*7. However, this service is only available to registered patients of virtual OPD / HIIMS.

Section - III

DTPA Scans of Patients Before and After GRAD system

Renal DTPA scan is a process for diagnosis and evaluation of kidney functioning to assess the drainage pattern of kidneys i.e., EGFR/ estimated glomerular filtration rate and is considered a GOLD STANDARD for assessing kidney function.

Find below the DTPA scans of some of the sample patients who followed GRAD System. Their renal scans clearly show the improvement.

Sample Patient-1 Before GRAD

Dated: 8 February 2022

Remarkable improvement seen with GRAD System just within 15 days even in failed transplant kidney

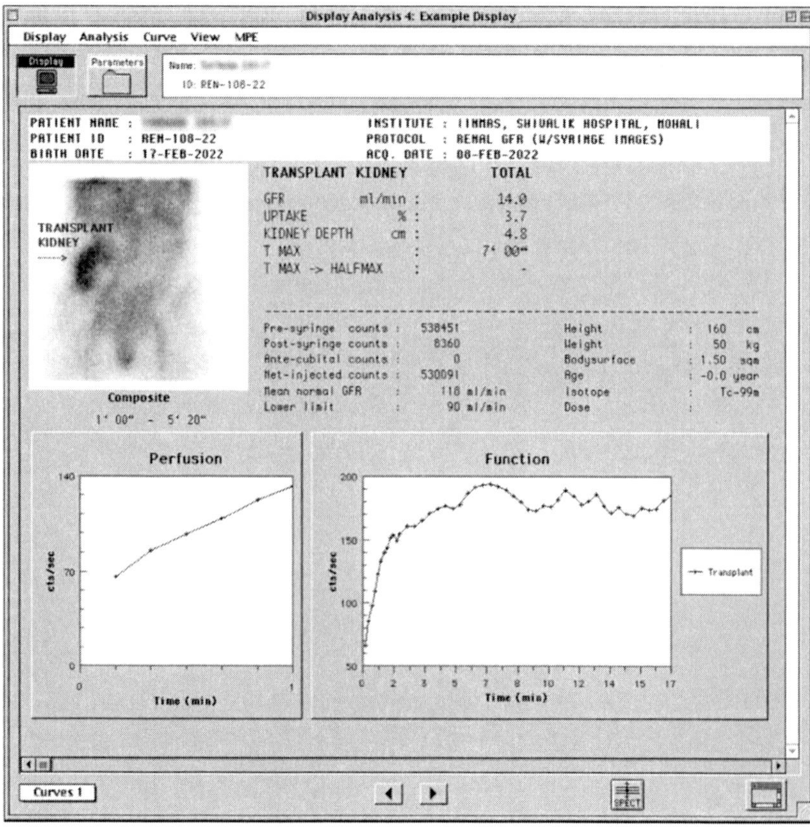

Sample Patient-1 Before GRAD

Dated: 8 February 2022

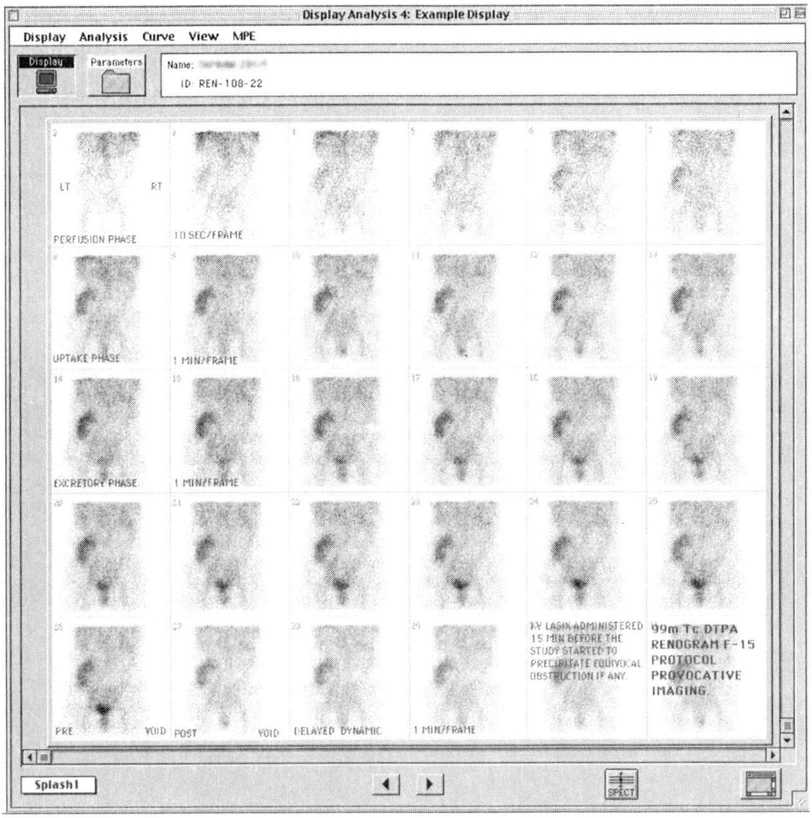

Sample Patient-1 After GRAD

Dated: 23 Feb 2022

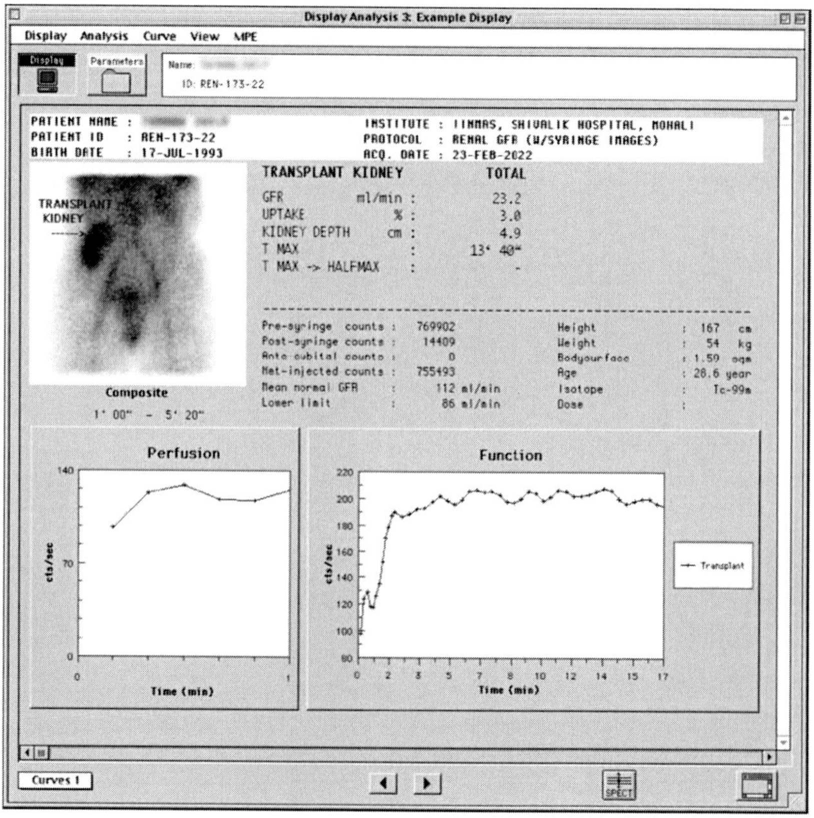

Sample Patient-1 After GRAD

Dated: 23 Feb 2022

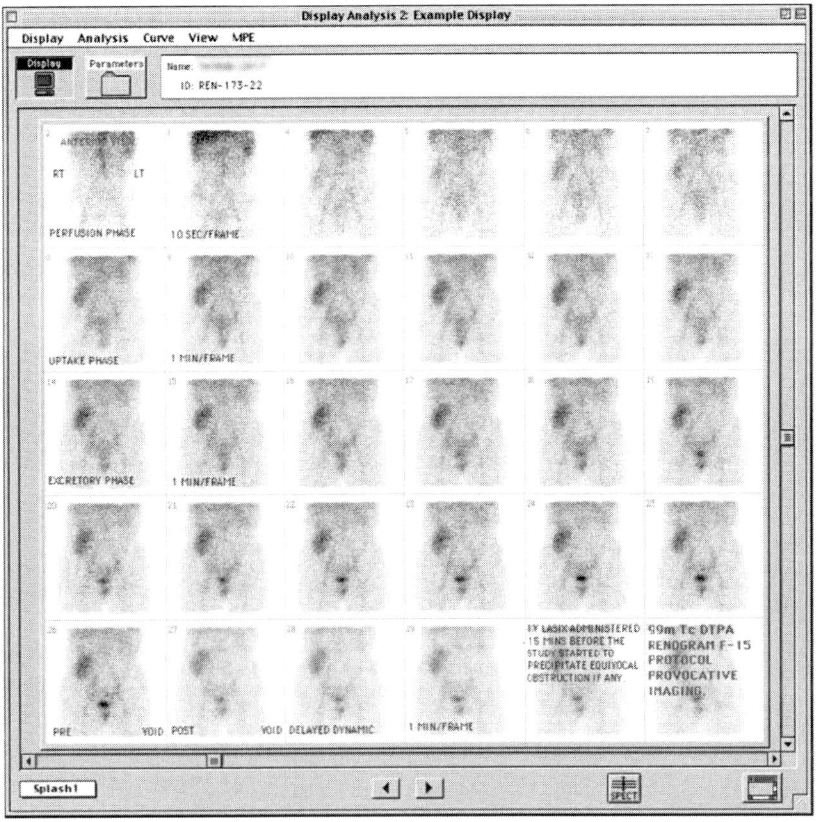

Sample Patient-2 Before GRAD

Dated: 11 November 2021

AERB Reg. No. 16-NMLICENSE-110822

INDIAN INSTITUTE OF NUCLEAR MEDICINE & SCANNING

Shivalik Hospital, Sector 69, Mohali,Ph. 0172-2216363, 5277528, 7009304465

Dr. AWADHESH PANDEY
Sr. Consultant & Head
Ex. FACULTY N.I.M.S. HYDERABAD

NAME : AGE : 14 Y SEX : F DATE: 11/11/2021
REG.NO. : REN-566-21
ATTENDING SR. PHYSICIAN: MANISH ACHARYA
CLINICAL STATUS: CKD, to know functional status, drainage pattern and AND differential function WITH GFR CALCULATION

DYNAMIC RENAL SCINTIGRAPHY

ISOTOPE: 99mTc- EC **DOSE: 5 mCi**

	LEFT KIDNEY	RIGHT KIDNEY
PERFUSION PHASE		
VISUALISATION	poor	poor
RELATIVE PERFUSION	poor	poor
UPTAKE PHASE		
SIZE	shrunk	shrunk
SHAPE	normal	normal
POSITION	normal	normal
CONCENTRATION	poor	poor
CORTICALMARGIN DELINEATION	poorly-defined	poorly defined
SPLIT FUNCTION	44 %	56 %
EXCRETORY PHASE		
COLLECTING SYSTEM	normal	normal
DRAINAGE PATTERN	normal	normal
DIURETIC RESPONSE	normal	normal
URETER	normal	normal
GFR	4.4 ml/min	5.6 ml/min

cont on page 2

NOT VALID FOR MEDICO-LEGAL PURPOSE

Sample Patient-2 Before GRAD

Dated: 11 November 2021

AERB Reg. No. 16-NMLICENSE-110822

INDIAN INSTITUTE OF NUCLEAR MEDICINE & SCANNING

Shivalik Hospital, Sector 69, Mohali,Ph. 0172-2216363, 5277528, 7009304465

Dr. AWADHESH PANDEY
Sr. Consultant & Head
Ex. FACULTY N.I.M.S. HYDERABAD

Page 2

IMPRESSION: PROVOCATIVE IMAGING WITH DIURETIC ADMINISTERED 15 MINUTES BEFORE THE STUDY, TO PRECIPITATE EQUIVOCAL OBSTRUCTION, IF ANY, REVEALS: -

LEFT KIDNEY i) SHRUNK IN SIZE
ii) SEVERELY COMPROMISED CORTICAL FUNCTION
iii) NORMAL DRAINAGE SEEN
a) improving on frusemide provocation
b) improving as a function of time

RIGHT KIDNEY i) SHRUNK IN SIZE
ii) SEVERELY COMPROMISED CORTICAL FUNCTION
iii) NORMAL DRAINAGE SEEN
a) improving on frusemide provocation
b) improving as a function of time

- GLOBAL GFR = 10.0 ml/min/1.15 sq m BSA
(normal range for BSA and age = 90 ml/min + - 17ml/min)

-SPLIT FUNCTION: LEFT KIDNEY = 44%
RIGHT KIDNEY = 56%

Awadhesh Pandey

Dr. AWADHESH PANDE Y
Sr. CONSULTANT & HEAD

NOT VALID FOR MEDICO-LEGAL PURPOSE

Sample Patient-2 Before GRAD

Dated: 11 November 2021

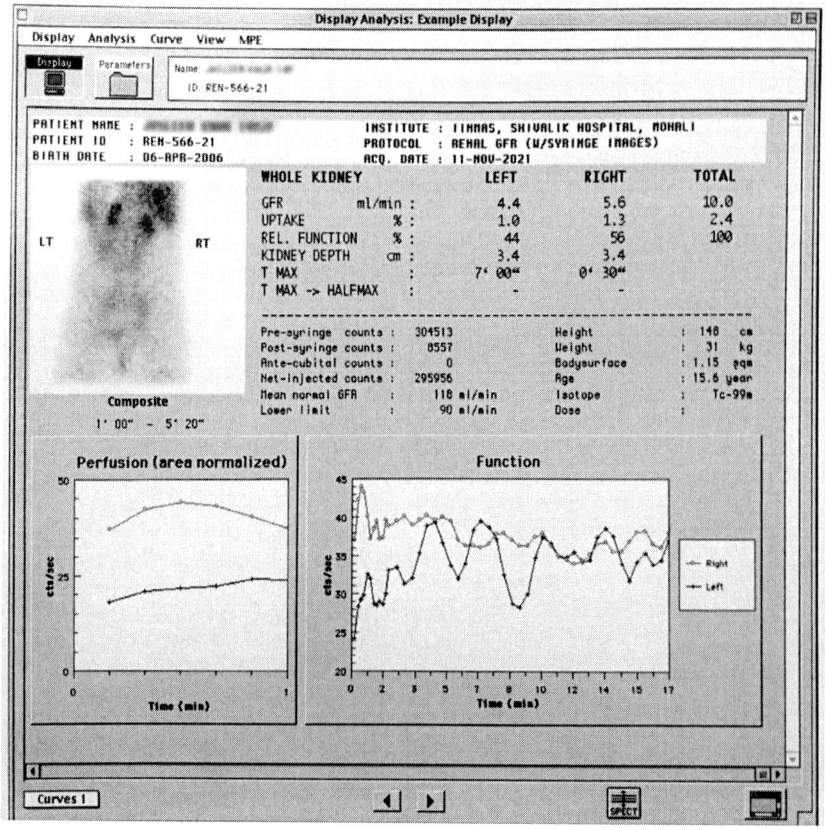

Sample Patient-2 Before GRAD

Dated: 11 November 2021

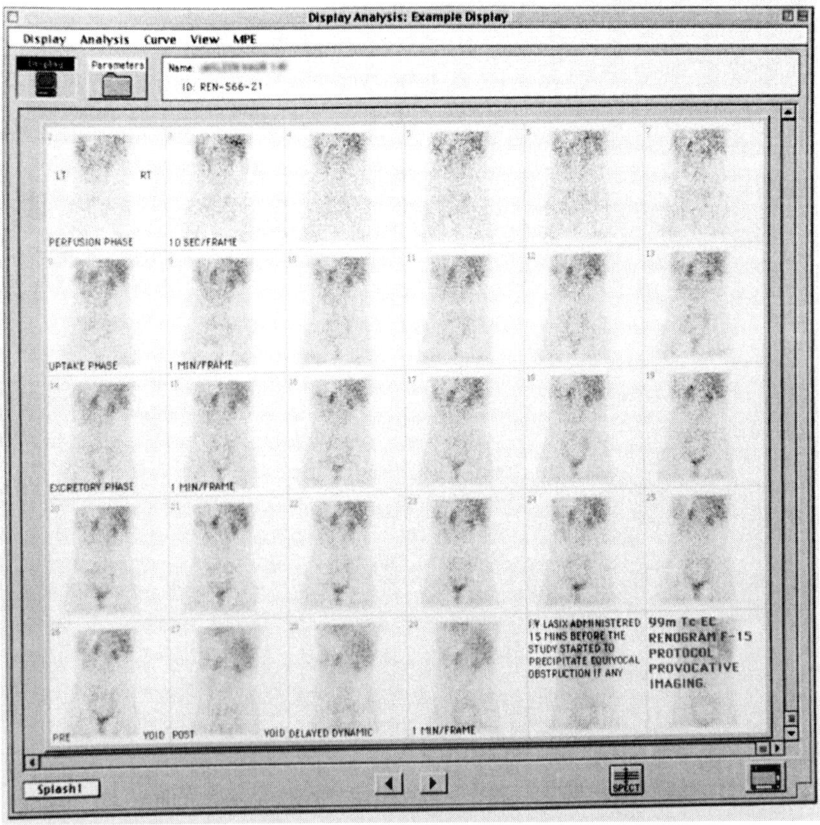

Sample Patient-2 After GRAD

Dated: 2 April 2022

AERB Reg. No. 16-NMLICENSE-110822

INDIAN INSTITUTE OF NUCLEAR MEDICINE & SCANNING

Shivalik Hospital, Sector 69, Mohali,Ph. 0172-2216363, 5277528, 7009304465

Dr. AWADHESH PANDEY
Sr. Consultant & Head
Ex. FACULTY N.I.M.S. HYDERABAD

NAME : [illegible] AGE : 14 Y SEX : F DATE: 02/04/2022
REG.NO. : REN-296-22
ATTENDING HOSPITAL: HIIMS, DERABASSI
CLINICAL STATUS: CKD, to know functional status, drainage pattern and AND differential function WITH GFR CALCULATION

DYNAMIC RENAL SCINTIGRAPHY

ISOTOPE: 99mTc- DTPA **DOSE: 5 mCi**

	LEFT KIDNEY	RIGHT KIDNEY
PERFUSION PHASE		
VISUALISATION	poor	poor
RELATIVE PERFUSION	poor	poor
UPTAKE PHASE		
SIZE	shrunk	shrunk
SHAPE	normal	normal
POSITION	normal	normal
CONCENTRATION	poor	poor
CORTICALMARGIN DELINEATION	poorly-defined	poorly defined
SPLIT FUNCTION	40 %	60 %
EXCRETORY PHASE		
COLLECTING SYSTEM	normal	normal
DRAINAGE PATTERN	normal	normal
DIURETIC RESPONSE	normal	normal
URETER	normal	normal
GFR	5.4 ml/min	8.2 ml/min

cont on page 2

NOT VALID FOR MEDICO-LEGAL PURPOSE

Sample Patient-2 After GRAD

Dated: 2 April 2022

AERB Reg. No. 16-NMLICENSE-110822

INDIAN INSTITUTE OF NUCLEAR MEDICINE & SCANNING

Shivalik Hospital, Sector 69, Mohali, Ph. 0172-2216363, 5277528, 7009304465

Dr. AWADHESH PANDEY
Sr. Consultant & Head
Ex. FACULTY N.I.M.S. HYDERABAD

Page 2

IMPRESSION: PROVOCATIVE IMAGING WITH DIURETIC ADMINISTERED 15 MINUTES BEFORE THE STUDY, TO PRECIPITATE EQUIVOCAL OBSTRUCTION, IF ANY, REVEALS: -

LEFT KIDNEY i) SHRUNK IN SIZE
ii) SEVERELY COMPROMISED CORTICAL FUNCTION
iii) NORMAL DRAINAGE SEEN
a) improving on frusemide provocation
b) improving as a function of time

RIGHT KIDNEY i) SHRUNK IN SIZE
ii) SEVERELY COMPROMISED CORTICAL FUNCTION
iii) NORMAL DRAINAGE SEEN
a) improving on frusemide provocation
b) improving as a function of time

- GLOBAL GFR = 13.7 ml/min/1.16 sq m BSA
(normal range for BSA and age = 90 ml/min + - 17ml/min)

-SPLIT FUNCTION: LEFT KIDNEY = 40 %
RIGHT KIDNEY = 60 %

N.B: AS COMPARED TO THE PREVIOUS SCAN DATED: 11 NOV 2021, THERE IS MILD IMPROVEMENT IN BILATERAL RENAL FUNCTION

Awadhesh Pandey

Dr. AWADHESH PANDE Y
Sr. CONSULTANT & HEAD

NOT VALID FOR MEDICO-LEGAL PURPOSE

Sample Patient-2 After GRAD

Dated: 2 April 2022

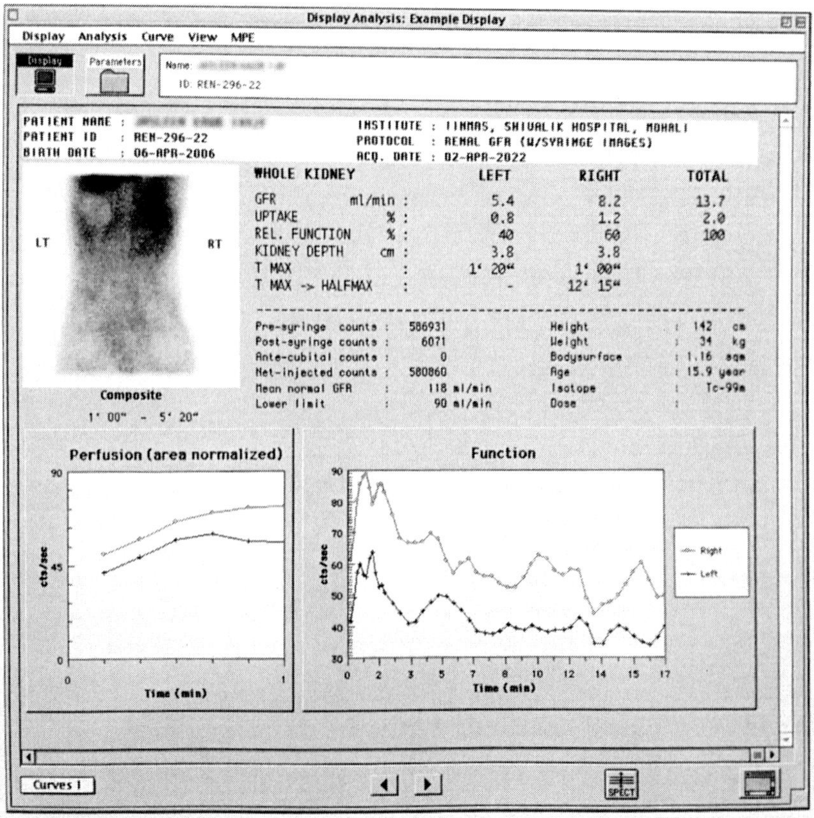

Sample Patient-2 After GRAD

Dated: 2 April 2022

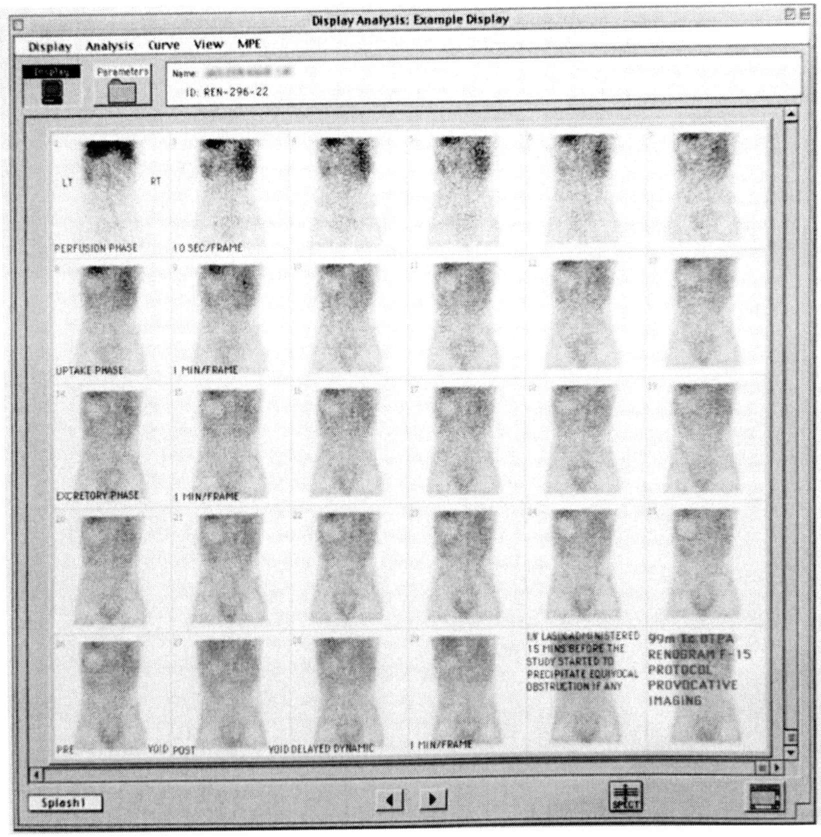

Sample Patient-3 Before GRAD

Dated : 27 November 2021

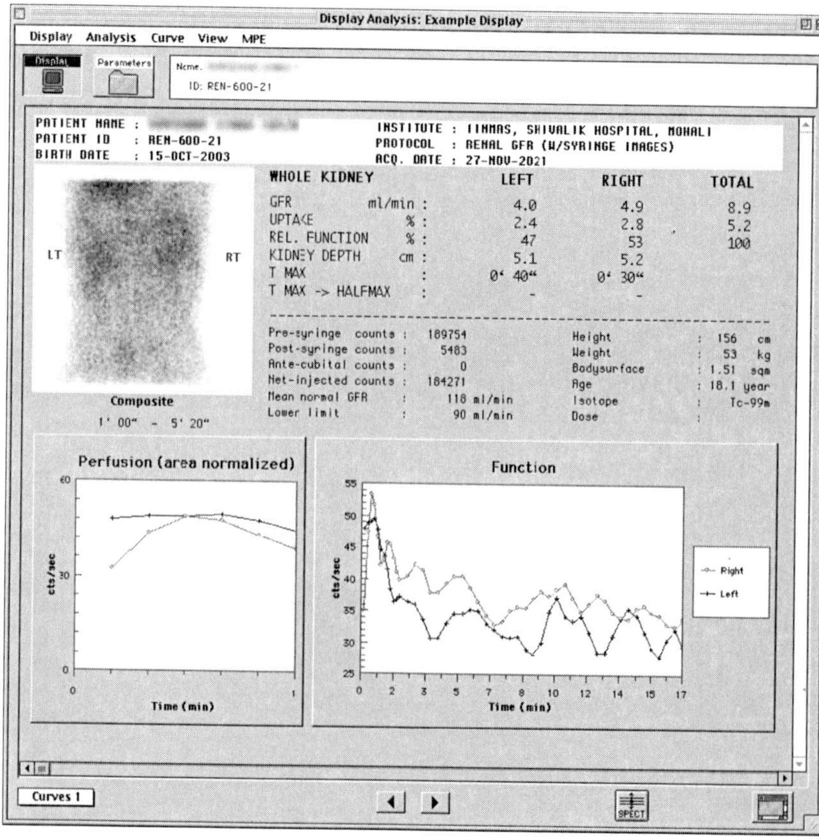

Sample Patient-3 Before GRAD

Dated : 27 November 2021

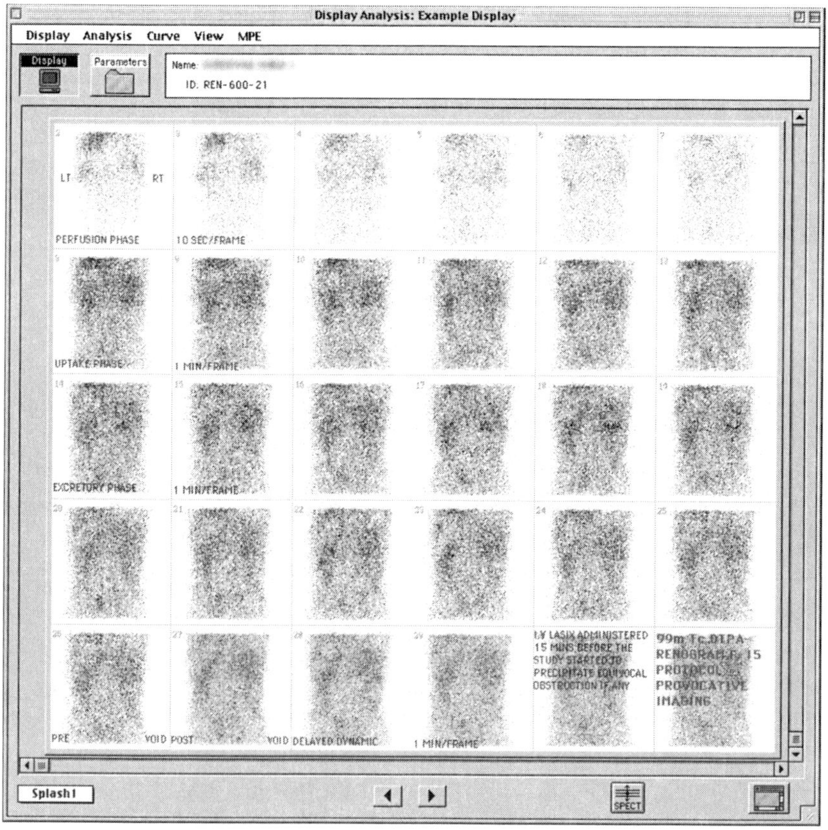

Sample Patient-3 After GRAD

Date: 21 February 2022

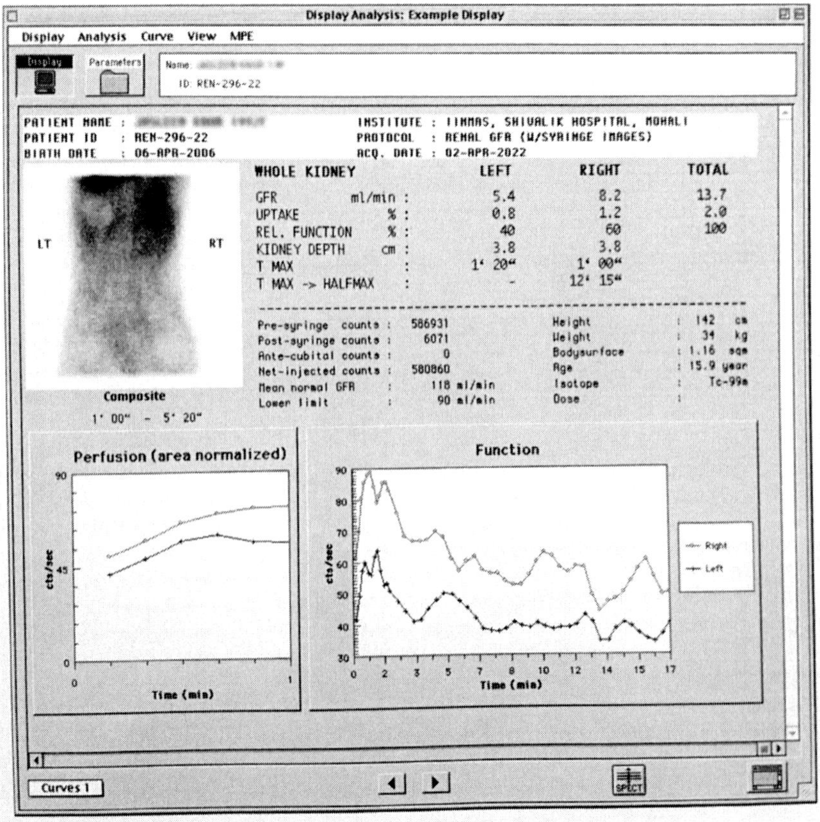

Sample Patient-3 After GRAD

Date: 21 February 2022

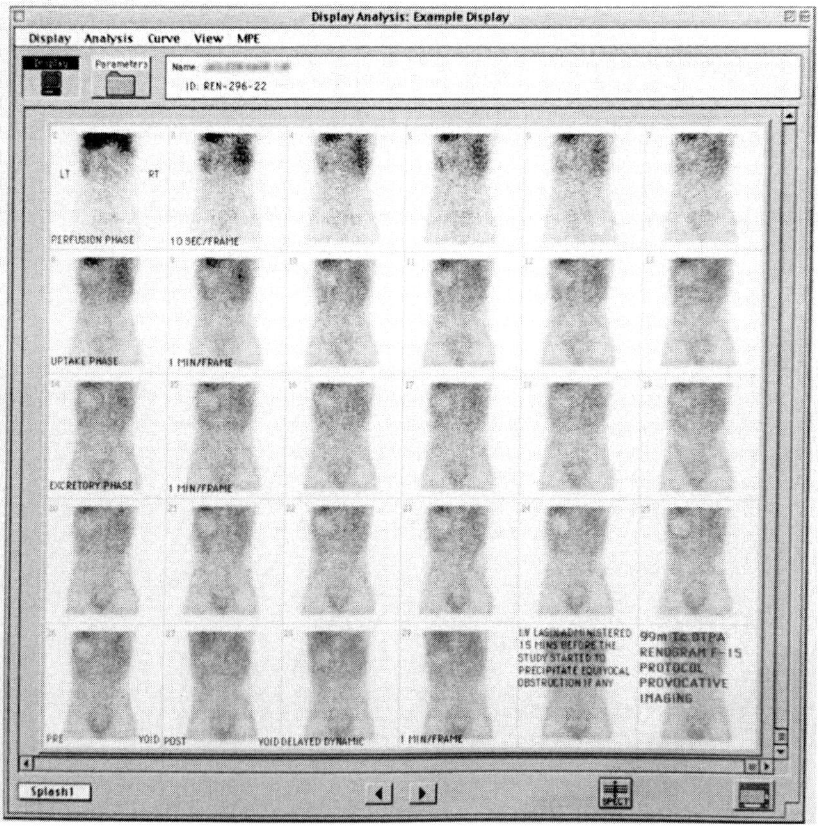

Sample Patient-4 Before GRAD

Dated : 4 June 2021

AERB Reg. No. 16-NMLICENSE-110822

INDIAN INSTITUTE OF NUCLEAR MEDICINE & SCANNING

Shivalik Hospital, Sector 69, Mohali,Ph. 0172-2216363, 5277528, 7009304465

Dr. AWADHESH PANDEY
Sr. Consultant & Head
Ex. FACULTY N.I.M.S. HYDERABAD

NAME: AGE: 65 Y SEX: M DATE: 04/06/2021
REG.NO. REN-279-21
ATTENDING SR. DOCTOR: ACHARYA MANISH
CLINICAL STATUS: TO KNOW FUNCTIONAL STATUS, GFR AND DRAINAGE PATTERN

DYNAMIC RENAL SCINTIGRAPHY
ISOTOPE: 99mTc-DTPA DOSE 5 m Ci

	LEFT KIDNEY	RIGHT KIDNEY
PERFUSION PHASE		
VISUALISATION	poor	poor
RELATIVE PERFUSION	poor	poor
UPTAKE PHASE		
SIZE	shrunk	shrunk
SHAPE	normal	normal
POSITION	normal	normal
CONCENTRATION	poor	poor
CORTICALMARGIN DELINEATION	poorly -defined	poorly-defined
SPLIT FUNCTION	45 %	55 %
EXCRETORY PHASE		
COLLECTING SYSTEM	normal	normal
DRAINAGE PATTERN	normal	normal
DIURETIC RESPONSE	normal	normal
URETER	normal	normal
GFR	6.5 ml/min	7.3 ml/min

CONT ON PG 2

Sample Patient-4 Before GRAD

Dated : 4 June 2021

AERB Reg. No. 16-NMLICENSE-110822

INDIAN INSTITUTE OF NUCLEAR MEDICINE & SCANNING

Shivalik Hospital, Sector 69, Mohali,Ph. 0172-2216363, 5277528, 7009304465

Dr. AWADHESH PANDEY
Sr. Consultant & Head
Ex. FACULTY N.I.M.S. HYDERABAD

Page 2

BLADDER: -NORMAL RESIDUAL VOLUME
-THERE IS NO DIFFRENCE IN TRACER CONCENTRATION BETWEEN
-PRE AND POST VOID FILMS SIGNIFYING NO INDIRECT EVIDENCE OF
i) VESICO-URETERIC REFLUX ON EITHER SIDE OR
ii) GRAVITY DEPENDENT DRAINAGE

IMPRESSION: PROVOCATIVE IMAGING WITH DIURETIC ADMINSISTERED 15 MINUTES BEFORE THE STUDY STARTED TO PRECIPITATE EQUIVOCAL OBSTRUCTION, IF ANY REVEALS:: -

LEFT KIDNEY i) SHRUNK IN SIZE
ii) SEVERELY COMPROMISED CORTICAL FUNCTION
iii) NORMAL DRAINAGE
I) improving on frusemide provocation
ii) improving as a function of time

RIGHT KIDNEY i) SHRUNK IN SIZE
ii) SEVERELY COMPROMISED CORTICAL FUNCTION
iii) NORMAL DRAINAGE
I) improving on frusemide provocation
ii) improving as a function of time

GLOBAL GFR = 13.8 ml/min/ 2.06 sq m BSA
(normal range for BSA = 73 ml/min + - 17ml/min)

SPLIT FUNCTION: LEFT KIDNEY = 45%
RIGHT KIDNEY = 55 %

Awadhesh Pandey

Dr.AWADHESH PANDEY
Sr.CONSULTANT & HEAD

END OF REPORT

Sample Patient-4 Before GRAD

Dated : 4 June 2021

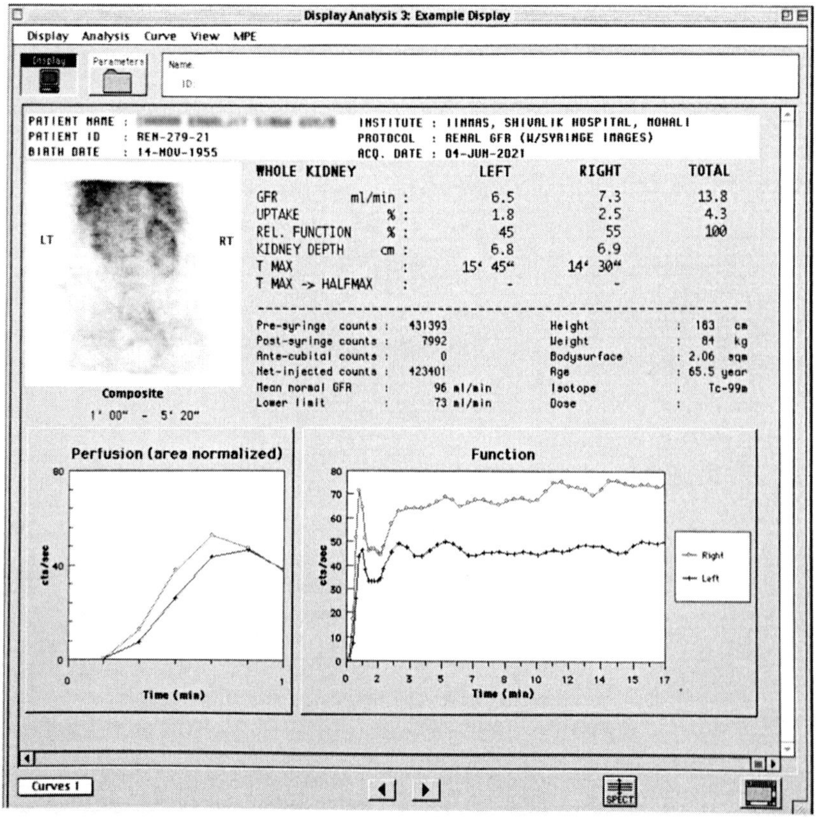

Sample Patient-4 Before GRAD

Dated : 4 June 2021

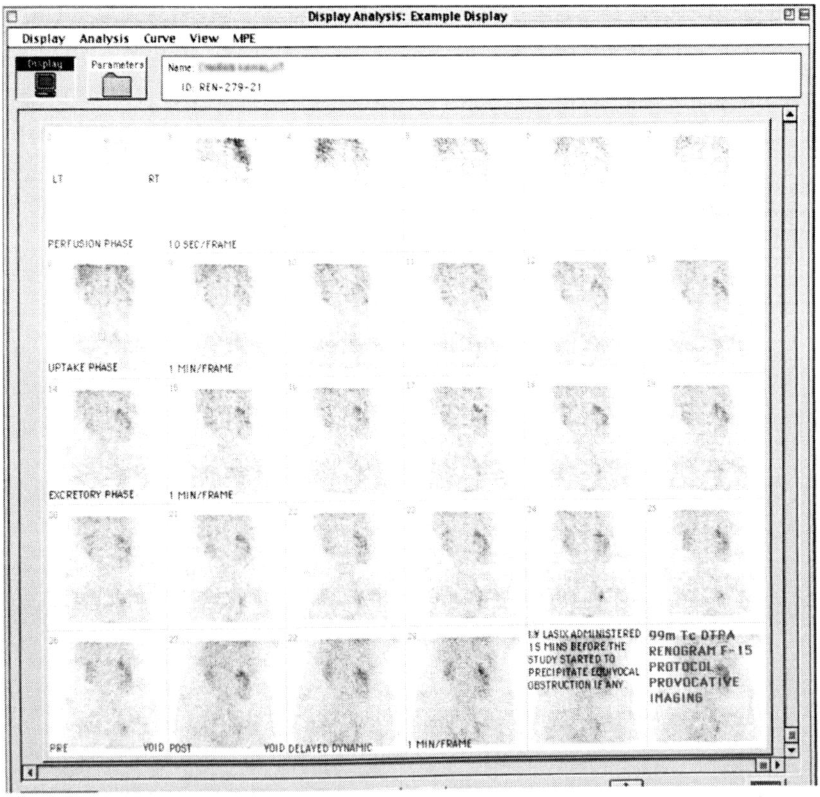

Sample Patient-4 After GRAD

Date: 27 August 2021

AERB Reg. No. 16-NMLICENSE-110822

INDIAN INSTITUTE OF NUCLEAR MEDICINE & SCANNING

Shivalik Hospital, Sector 69, Mohali, Ph. 0172-2216363, 5277528, 7009304465

Dr. AWADHESH PANDEY
Sr. Consultant & Head
Ex. FACULTY N.I.M.S. HYDERABAD

NAME : [illegible] AGE : 65 Y SEX : M DATE: 27/08/2021
REG.NO. : REN-444-21
ATTENDING SR. PHYSICIAN: MANISH ACHARYA
CLINICAL STATUS: CKD, to know functional status, drainage pattern and AND differential function WITH GFR

DYNAMIC RENAL SCINTIGRAPHY

ISOTOPE: 99mTc- DTPA **DOSE: 5 mCi**

	LEFT KIDNEY	RIGHT KIDNEY
PERFUSION PHASE		
VISUALISATION	poor	poor
RELATIVE PERFUSION	poor	poor
UPTAKE PHASE		
SIZE	shrunk	shrunk
SHAPE	normal	normal
POSITION	normal	normal
CONCENTRATION	poor	poor
CORTICALMARGIN DELINEATION	poorly-defined	poorly defined
SPLIT FUNCTION	42 %	58 %
EXCRETORY PHASE		
COLLECTING SYSTEM	normal	normal
DRAINAGE PATTERN	normal	normal
DIURETIC RESPONSE	normal	normal
URETER	normal	normal
GFR	8.0 ml/min	10.8 ml/min

cont on page 2

Sample Patient-4 After GRAD

Date: 27 August 2021

AERB Reg. No. 16-NMLICENSE-110822

INDIAN INSTITUTE OF NUCLEAR MEDICINE & SCANNING

Shivalik Hospital, Sector 69, Mohali, Ph. 0172-2216363, 5277528, 7009304465

Dr. AWADHESH PANDEY
Sr. Consultant & Head
Ex. FACULTY N.I.M.S. HYDERABAD

Page 2

IMPRESSION: PROVOCATIVE IMAGING WITH DIURETIC ADMINISTERED 15 MINUTES BEFORE THE STUDY, TO PRECIPITATE EQUIVOCAL OBSTRUCTION, IF ANY, REVEALS: -

LEFT KIDNEY i) SHRUNK IN SIZE
ii) SEVERELY COMPROMISED CORTICAL FUNCTION
iii) NORMAL DRAINAGE SEEN
a) improving on frusemide provocation
b) improving as a function of time

RIGHT KIDNEY i) SHRUNK IN SIZE
ii) SEVERELY COMPROMISED CORTICAL FUNCTION
iii) NORMAL DRAINAGE SEEN
a) improving on frusemide provocation
b) improving as a function of time

- GLOBAL GFR = 18.8 ml/min/2.03 sq m BSA
(normal range for BSA and age = 73 ml/min + - 17ml/min)

-SPLIT FUNCTION: LEFT KIDNEY = 42%
RIGHT KIDNEY = 58%

N.B: AS COMPARED TO THE PREVIOUS SCAN DATED: 04 JUNE 2021, THERE IS IMPROVEMENT IN BILATERAL RENAL FUNCTION AND GFR

Awadhesh Pandey

Dr. AWADHESH PANDE Y
Sr. CONSULTANT & HEAD

Sample Patient-4 After GRAD

Date: 27 August 2021

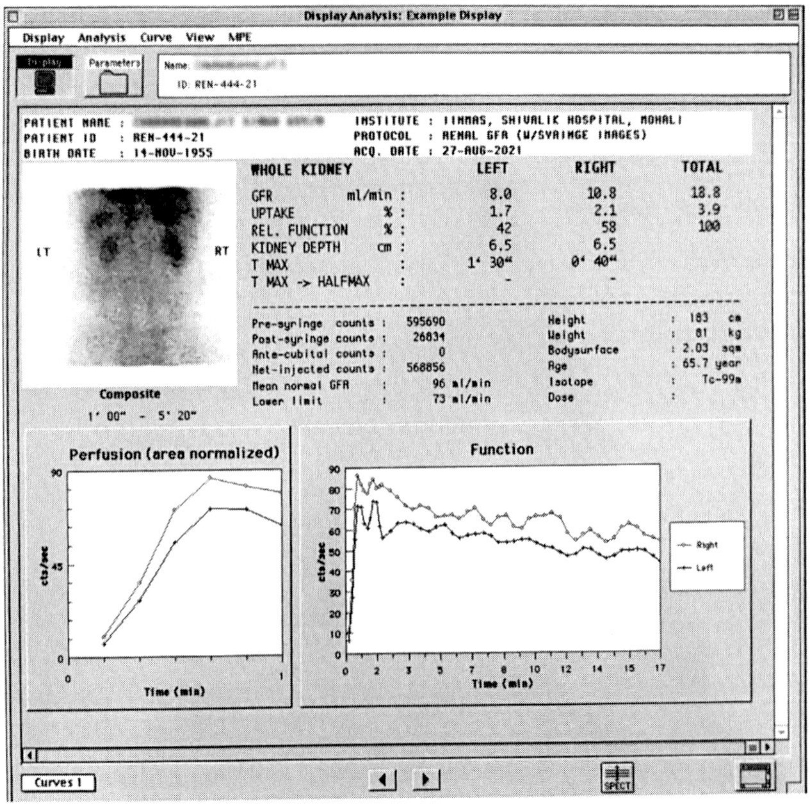

Sample Patient-4 After GRAD

Date: 27 August 2021

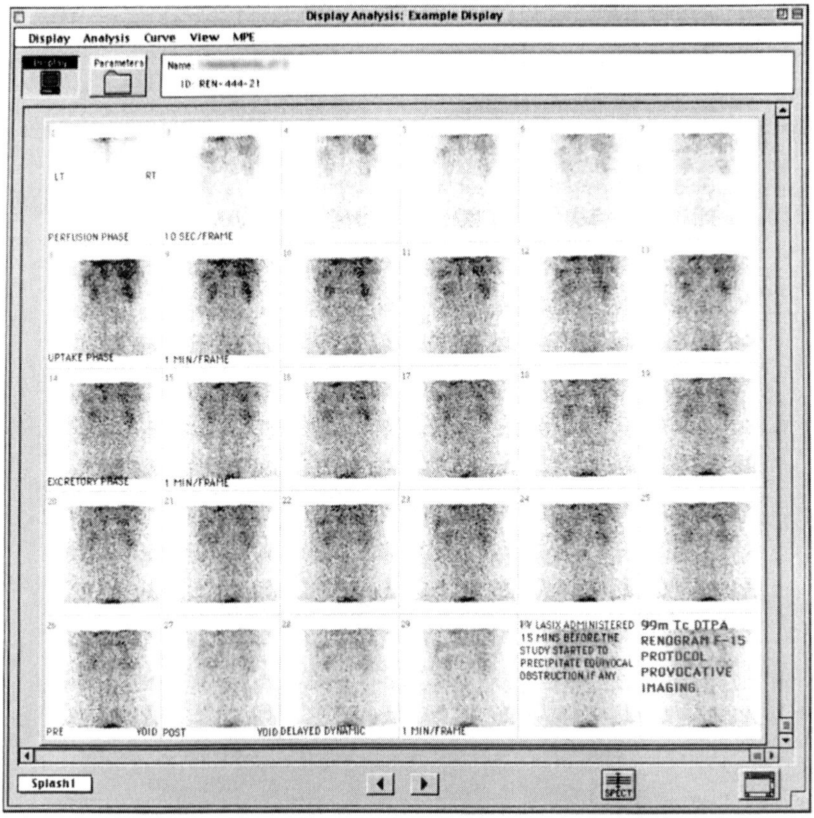

Sample Patient-5 Before GRAD

Dated : 7 January 2022

NAME : [illegible] AGE : 36 Y SEX : M DATE: 07/01/2022
REG.NO. : REN-09-22
ATTENDING HOSPITAL: HIIMS, DERABASSI
CLINICAL STATUS: CKD, to know functional status, drainage pattern and AND differential function WITH GFR CALCULATION

DYNAMIC RENAL SCINTIGRAPHY

ISOTOPE: 99mTc- DTPA **DOSE: 5 mCi**

	LEFT KIDNEY	RIGHT KIDNEY
PERFUSION PHASE		
VISUALISATION	poor	poor
RELATIVE PERFUSION	poor	poor
UPTAKE PHASE		
SIZE	shrunk	shrunk
SHAPE	normal	normal
POSITION	normal	normal
CONCENTRATION	poor	poor
CORTICALMARGIN DELINEATION	poorly-defined	poorly defined
SPLIT FUNCTION	50%	50%
EXCRETORY PHASE		
COLLECTING SYSTEM	normal	normal
DRAINAGE PATTERN	normal	normal
DIURETIC RESPONSE	normal	normal
URETER	normal	normal
GFR	4.0 ml/min	4.0 ml/min

cont on page 2

Sample Patient-5 Before GRAD

Dated : 7 January 2022

Page 2

IMPRESSION: PROVOCATIVE IMAGING WITH DIURETIC ADMINISTERED 15 MINUTES BEFORE THE STUDY, TO PRECIPITATE EQUIVOCAL OBSTRUCTION, IF ANY, REVEALS: -

LEFT KIDNEY i) **SHRUNK IN SIZE**
ii) SEVERELY COMPROMISED CORTICAL FUNCTION
iii) NORMAL DRAINAGE SEEN
a) improving **on frusemide provocation**
b) improving **as a function of time**

RIGHT KIDNEY i) **SHRUNK IN SIZE**
ii) SEVERELY COMPROMISED CORTICAL FUNCTION
iii) NORMAL DRAINAGE SEEN
a) improving **on frusemide provocation**
b) improving **as a function of time**

- GLOBAL GFR = 8.0 ml/min/1.69 sq m BSA
(normal range for BSA and age = 84 ml/min + - 17ml/min)

-SPLIT FUNCTION: LEFT KIDNEY = **50%**
RIGHT KIDNEY = **50%**

N.B: PLEASE RULE OUT ESRD (END STAGE RENAL DISEASE)

REPEAT DTPA SCAN AFTER 3 MONTHS TO SEE PROGRESSION OR REGRESSION

Dr. AWADHESH PANDE Y
Sr. CONSULTANT & HEAD

Sample Patient-5 Before GRAD

Dated : 7 January 2022

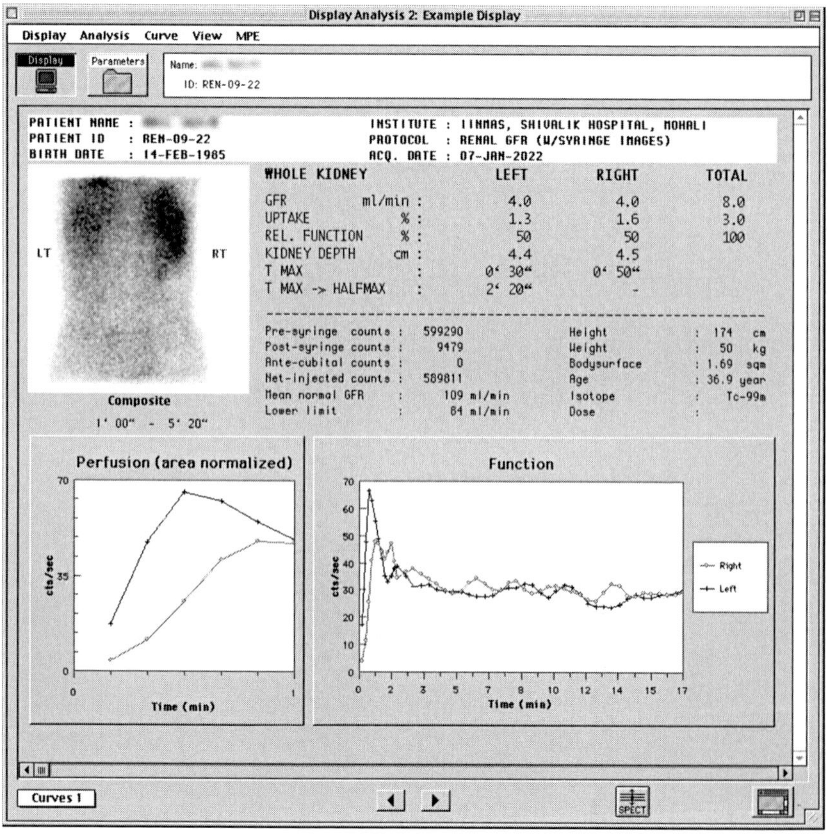

Sample Patient-5 Before GRAD

Dated : 7 January 2022

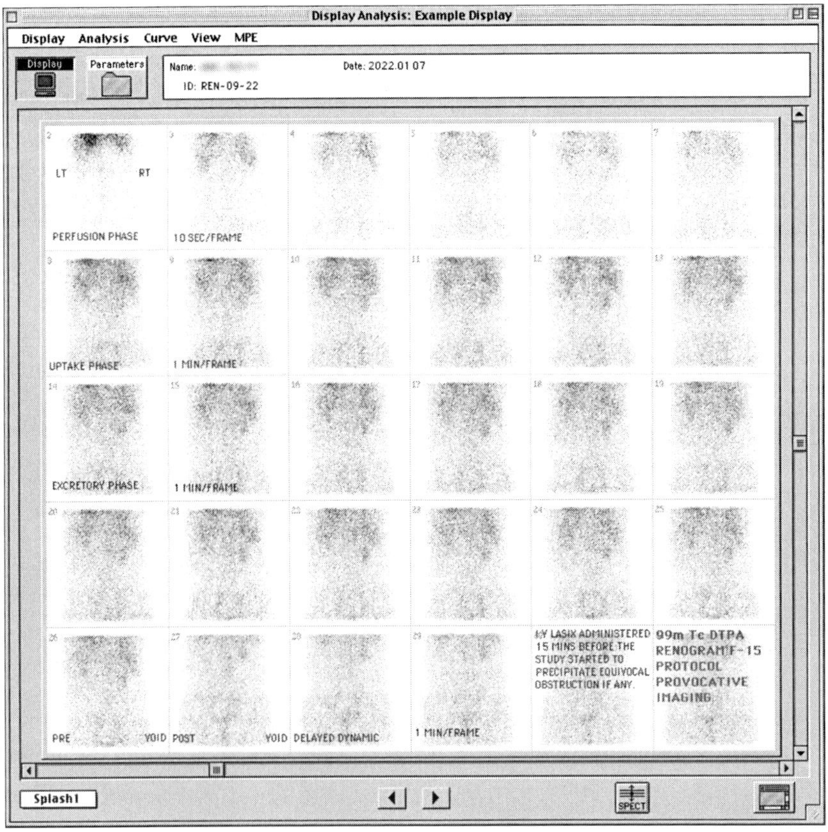

Sample Patient-5 After GRAD

Date: 26 April 2022

NAME : [illegible] AGE : 37 Y SEX : M DATE: 26/04/2022
REG.NO. : REN-362-22
ATTENDING HOSPITAL: HIIMS, DERABASSI
CLINICAL STATUS: CKD, to know functional status, drainage pattern and AND differential function WITH GFR CALCULATION

DYNAMIC RENAL SCINTIGRAPHY

ISOTOPE: 99mTc- DTPA DOSE: 5 mCi

	LEFT KIDNEY	RIGHT KIDNEY
PERFUSION PHASE		
VISUALISATION	poor	poor
RELATIVE PERFUSION	poor	poor
UPTAKE PHASE		
SIZE	shrunk	shrunk
SHAPE	normal	normal
POSITION	normal	normal
CONCENTRATION	poor	poor
CORTICALMARGIN DELINEATION	poorly-defined	poorly defined
SPLIT FUNCTION	47 %	53 %
EXCRETORY PHASE		
COLLECTING SYSTEM	normal	normal
DRAINAGE PATTERN	normal	normal
DIURETIC RESPONSE	normal	normal
URETER	normal	normal
GFR	7.5 ml/min	8.0 ml/min

cont on page 2

Sample Patient-5 After GRAD

Date: 26 April 2022

Page 2

IMPRESSION: PROVOCATIVE IMAGING WITH DIURETIC ADMINISTERED 15 MINUTES BEFORE THE STUDY, TO PRECIPITATE EQUIVOCAL OBSTRUCTION, IF ANY, REVEALS: -

LEFT KIDNEY i) **SHRUNK IN SIZE**
ii) SEVERELY COMPROMISED CORTICAL FUNCTION
iii) NORMAL DRAINAGE SEEN
a) improving **on frusemide provocation**
b) improving **as a function of time**

RIGHT KIDNEY i) **SHRUNK IN SIZE**
ii) SEVERELY COMPROMISED CORTICAL FUNCTION
iii) NORMAL DRAINAGE SEEN
a) improving **on frusemide provocation**
b) improving **as a function of time**

- GLOBAL GFR = 15.5 ml/min/1.59 sq m BSA
(normal range for BSA and age = 84 ml/min + - 17ml/min)

-SPLIT FUNCTION: LEFT KIDNEY = **47 %**
RIGHT KIDNEY = **53 %**

N.B: AS COMPARED TO THE PREVIOUS SCAN DATED: 07 JAN 2022, THERE IS IMPROVEMENT IN BILATERAL RENAL FUNCTION

Awadhesh Pandey

Dr. AWADHESH PANDE Y
Sr. CONSULTANT & HEAD

Sample Patient-5 After GRAD

Date: 26 April 2022

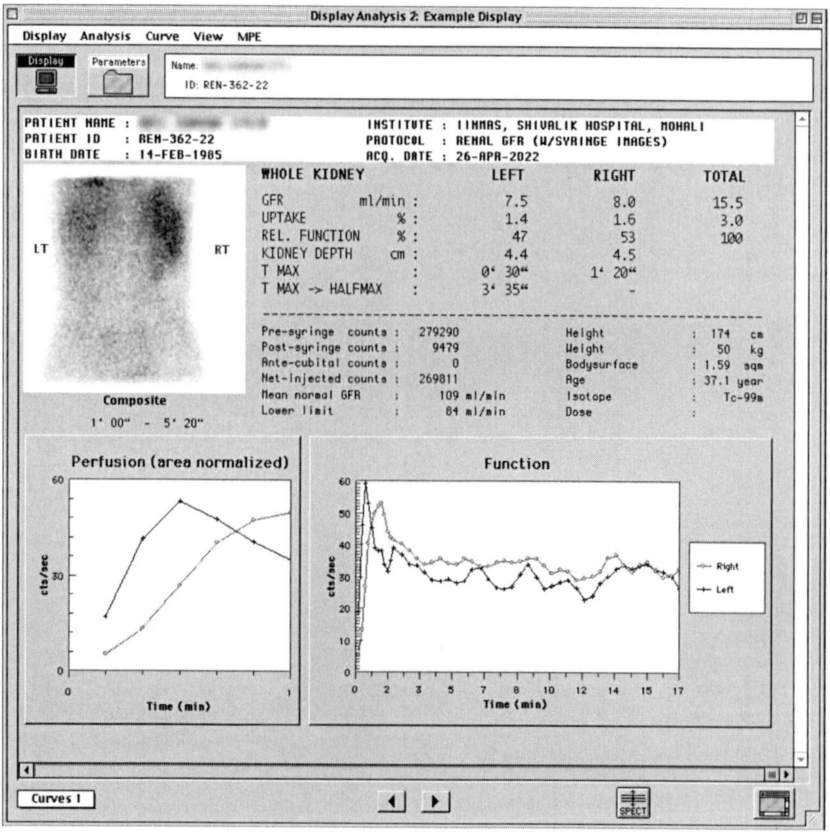

Sample Patient-5 After GRAD

Date: 26 April 2022

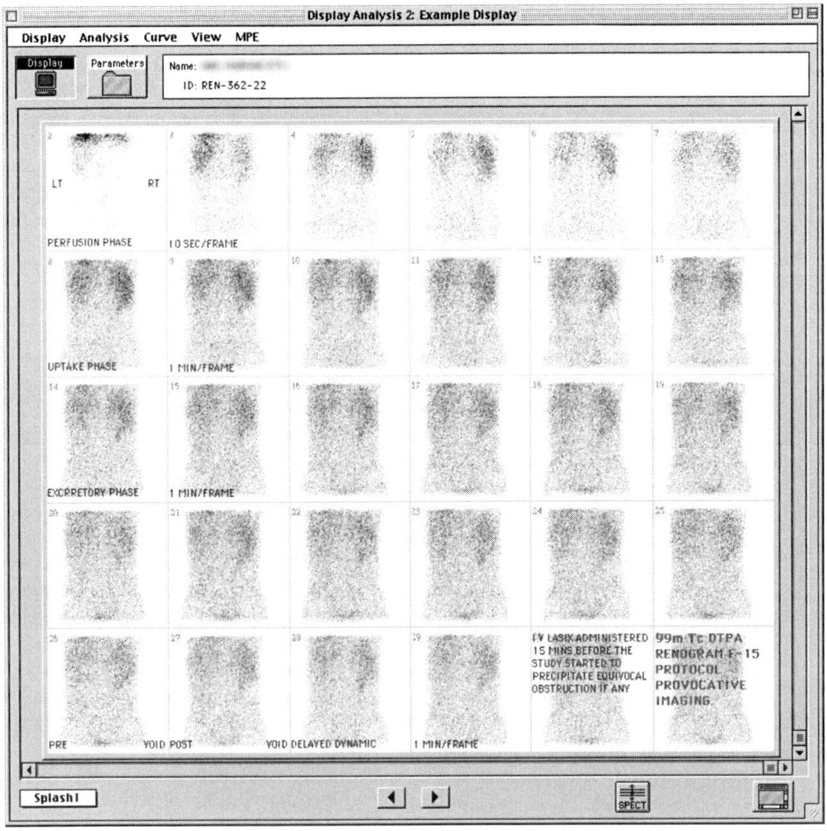

Sample Patient-6 Before GRAD

Dated: 12 January 2022

NAME: [illegible] AGE: 24Y SEX M DATE- 12/01/2022
REG.NO. 438932
CLINICAL STATUS: To Access Functional status, Drainage pattern

PROVOCATIVE DYNAMIC RENAL SCINTIGRAPHY
ISOTOPE: 99mTc-DTPA DOSE : 5 m Ci

	LEFT KIDNEY	RIGHT KIDNEY
PERFUSION PHASE		
VISUALISATION	poor	poor
RELATIVE PERFUSION	poor	poor
UPTAKE PHASE		
SIZE	shrunk	shrunk
SHAPE	normal	normal
POSITION	normal	normal
CONCENTRATION	poor	poor
CORTICALMARGIN DELINEATION	poorly -defined	poorlly-defined
SPLIT FUNCTION	39.5%	60.5%
EXCRETORY PHASE		
COLLECTING SYSTEM	normal	normal
DRAINAGE PATTERN	normal	normal
DIURETIC RESPONSE	normal	normal
URETER	normal	normal
GFR	0.155ml/min	0.236 ml/min

--------------------CONT ON PG 2--------------------

Page 2

Sample Patient-6 Before GRAD

Dated: 12 January 2022

BLADDER: - NORMAL RESIDUAL VOLUME
-THERE IS DIFFRENCE IN TRACER CONCENTRATION BETWEEN
-PRE AND POST VOID FILMS SIGNIFYING INDIRECT EVIDENCE OF
i VESICO-URETERIC REFLUX ON RIGHT SIDE.

IMPRESSION:PROVOCATIVE IMAGING WITH DIURETIC ADMINSISTERED 15 MINUTES BEFORE THE STUDY STARTED TO PRECIPITATE EQUIVOCAL OBSTRUCTION, IF ANY REVEALS: -

LEFT KIDNEY i SHRUNK IN SIZE
ii) SEVERELY COMPROMISED CORTICAL FUNCTION
iii) NORMAL DRAINAGE

RIGHT KIDNEY i SHRUNK IN SIZE
ii) SEVERELY COMPROMISED CORTICAL FUNCTION
iii) NORMAL DRAINAGE

- GLOBAL GFR = 0.391ml/min/ sq m BSA
(normal range for BSA = 90 ml/min + - 17ml/min)

-SPLIT FUNCTION: LEFT KIDNEY = 39.5%
RIGHT KIDNEY = 60.5 %

NB- PLEASE RULE OUT END STAGE RENAL DISEASE

Dr.AWADHESH PANDE Y
Sr.CONSULTANT & HEAD

END OF REPORT

Sample Patient-6 Before GRAD

Dated: 12 January 2022

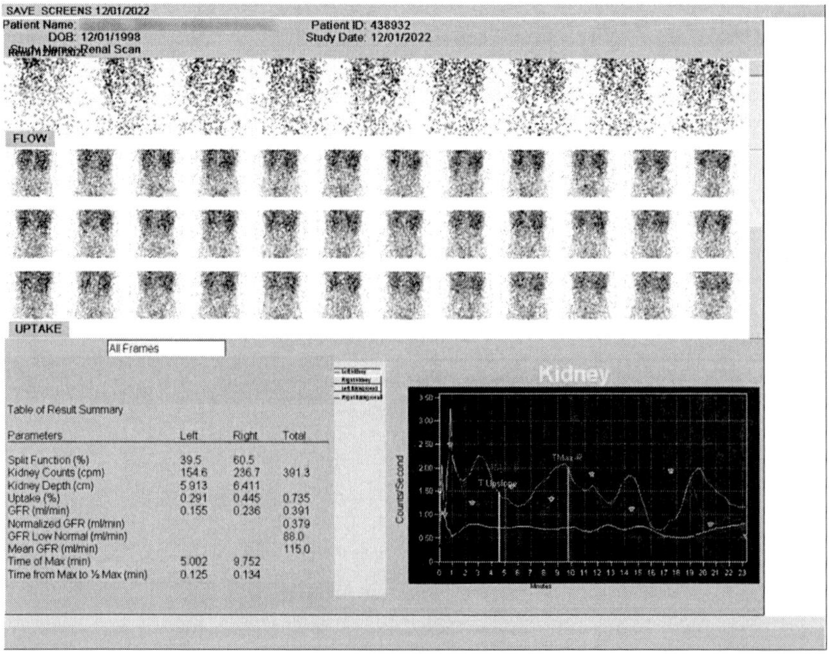

Table of Result Summary

Parameters	Left	Right	Total
Split Function (%)	39.5	60.5	
Kidney Counts (cpm)	154.6	236.7	391.3
Kidney Depth (cm)	5.913	6.411	
Uptake (%)	0.291	0.445	0.735
GFR (ml/min)	0.155	0.236	0.391
Normalized GFR (ml/min)			0.379
GFR Low Normal (ml/min)			88.0
Mean GFR (ml/min)			115.0
Time of Max (min)	5.002	9.752	
Time from Max to ½ Max (min)	0.125	0.134	

Sample Patient-6 After GRAD

Dated: 18 April 2022

NAME: [illegible] AGE: 25Y SEX M DATE: 18/04/2022
REG.NO. 438932
CLINICAL STATUS: To Know FUNCTIONAL STATUS, DRAINAGE PATTERN, SPLIT FUNCTION, AND GFR

PROVOCATIVE DYNAMIC RENAL SCINTIGRAPHY

ISOTOPE: 99mTc-DTPA DOSE : 5 m Ci

	LEFT KIDNEY	RIGHT KIDNEY
PERFUSION PHASE		
VISUALISATION	poor	poor
RELATIVE PERFUSION	poor	poor
UPTAKE PHASE		
SIZE	shrunk	shrunk
SHAPE	normal	normal
POSITION	normal	normal
CONCENTRATION	poor	poor
CORTICALMARGIN DELINEATION	poorly-defined	poorly-defined
SPLIT FUNCTION	34.6%	65.4%
EXCRETORY PHASE		
COLLECTING SYSTEM	normal	normal
DRAINAGE PATTERN	normal	normal
DIURETIC RESPONSE	normal	normal
URETER	normal	normal
GFR	3.221ml/min	6.085 ml/min

CONT ON PG 2

Sample Patient-6 After GRAD

Dated: 18 April 2022

Page 2

BLADDER: - NORMAL RESIDUAL VOLUME
-THERE IS NO DIFFRENCE IN TRACER CONCENTRATION BETWEEN
-PRE AND POST VOID FILMS SIGNIFYING NO INDIRECT EVIDENCE OF
i i) VESICO-URETERIC REFLUX ON EITHER SIDE OR
ii ii) GRAVITY DEPENDENT DRAINAGE.

IMPRESSION: - 99m Tc DTPA RENOGRAM REVEALS: -

LEFT KIDNEY i) SHRUNK IN SIZE
ii) SEVERELY COPROMISED CORTICAL FUNCTION
iii) THERE IS EVIDENCE OF NORMAL DRAINAGE
a) improving on frusemide provocation
b) improving as a function of time

RIGHT KIDNEY i) SHRUNK IN SIZE
ii) SEVERELY COMPROMISED CORTICAL FUNCTION
iii) THERE IS EVIDENCE OF NORMAL DRAINAGE
a) improving on frusemide provocation
b) improving as a function of time

- GLOBAL GFR = 9.306ml/min/sq m BSA
(normal range for BSA = 73ml/min + - 17ml/min)

-SPLIT FUNCTION: LEFT KIDNEY = 34.6%
RIGHT KIDNEY = 65.4%

NB- AS COMPARE TO PREVIOUS STUDY (12/01/2022) THERE IS IMPROVEMENT IN BILATERAL RENAL FUNCTION

Awadhesh Pandey

Dr.AWADHESH PANDEY
Sr.CONSULTANT & HEAD

END OF REPORT

Sample Patient-6 After GRAD

Dated: 18 April 2022

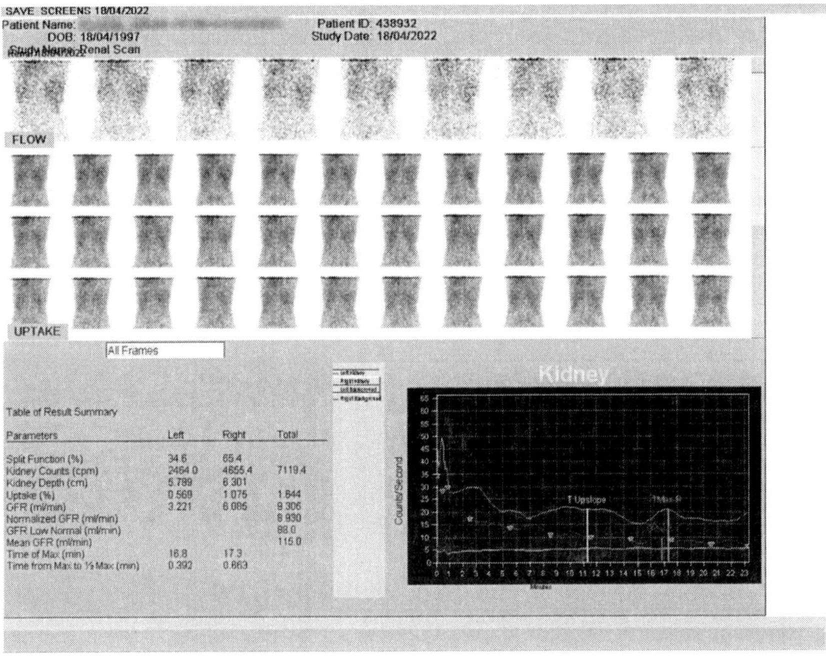

Table of Result Summary

Parameters	Left	Right	Total
Split Function (%)	34.6	65.4	
Kidney Counts (cpm)	2464.0	4655.4	7119.4
Kidney Depth (cm)	5.789	6.301	
Uptake (%)	0.568	1.075	1.644
GFR (ml/min)	3.221	6.085	9.306
Normalized GFR (ml/min)			8.930
GFR Low Normal (ml/min)			88.0
Mean GFR (ml/min)			115.0
Time of Max (min)	16.8	17.3	
Time from Max to ½ Max (min)	0.392	0.863	

Sample Patient-7 Before GRAD

Dated: 15 December 2021

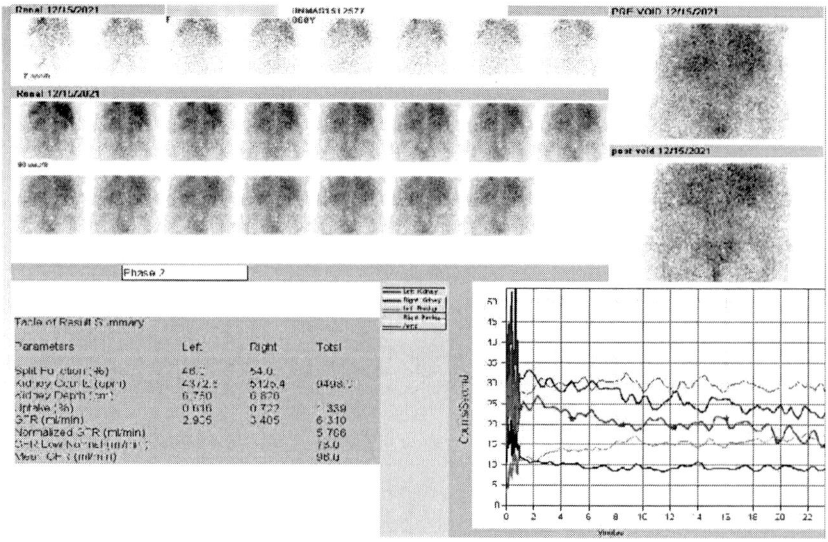

Sample Patient-7 After GRAD

Dated: 29 March 2022

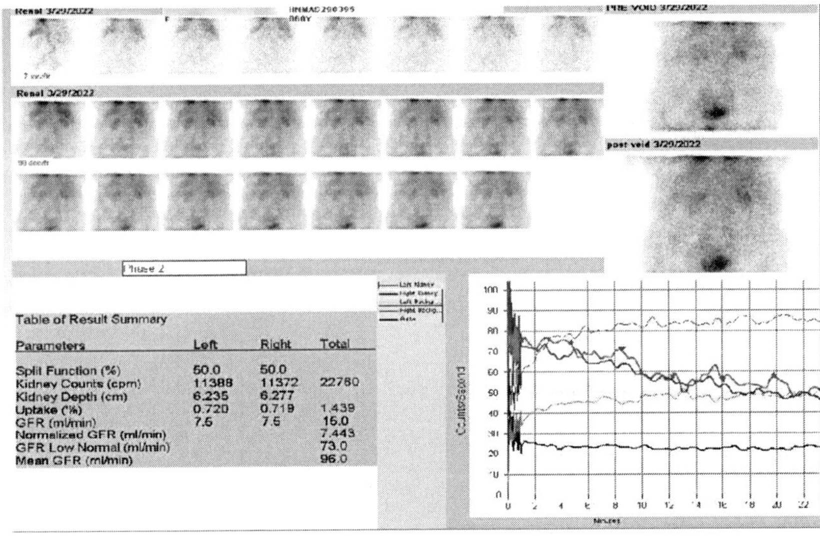

Table of Result Summary

Parameters	Left	Right	Total
Split Function (%)	50.0	50.0	
Kidney Counts (cpm)	11388	11372	22760
Kidney Depth (cm)	6.235	6.277	
Uptake (%)	0.720	0.719	1.439
GFR (ml/min)	7.5	7.5	15.0
Normalized GFR (ml/min)			7.443
GFR Low Normal (ml/min)			73.0
Mean GFR (ml/min)			96.0

Health Freedom
with
N.I.C.E & W.I.S.E

Dr. Biswaroop Roy Chowdhury and his N.I.C.E (Network of Influenza Ca Experts) team have helped and cured more than 50,000 COVID-19 an other infectious/communicable diseases patients (including smallpo typhoid, tuberculosis) with zero medicine / money / mortality.

Now health freedom through W.I.S.E (Wellness and Inflammator Syndrome Experts) for more than 60 types of non-communicable / lifesty illnesses.

Service to the Nation in 2 Steps

Step-1: Call our 24x7 helpline number: +91-8587059169.

Step-2: Fill the details of the patient in the link given below.

www.biswaroop.com/nice
(Influenza/Communicable diseases)

www.biswaroop.com/wise
(Lifestyle/Non-communicable diseases)

N.I.C.E

W.I.S.E

Let every morning be the Hunza Morning

If you have decided to pick only one of my suggestions for the sake of your health, then take this suggestion :

Stop consuming tea specially, morning tea. The early morning tea makes the inner lining of your intestinal wall acidic, as after a long night of fasting your stomach is empty and craving for food. An acidic stomach on a regular basis is the single biggest cause of all kind of inflammatory and lifestyle diseases including arthritis, Diabetes etc.

How to stop craving of tea ⟶ Switch to Hunza Tea

Hunza Civilization: Hunza people are the Indians living at extreme northwest of India in Hindu Kush range. They are known to be one of the world's healthiest civilizations, often living up to the age of 110 years.

How to prepare Hunza Tea (serves four):

Ingredients:

- 12 Mint leaves(Pudina)
- 8 Basil Leaves(Tulsi)
- 4 Green cardamom (Elaichi)
- 2 gm Cinnamon (Dalchini)
- 20 gm Ginger (Adrak)
- 20 gm Jaggery (Gur)

Instructions:

- Take 4 cups of water in a tea pan
- Add all ingredients, simmer it for 10mins
- Add a dash of lemon juice and serve hot or cold